Metabolic Aspects of PCOS

Mariagrazia Stracquadanio • Lilliana Ciotta

Metabolic Aspects of PCOS

Treatment with Insulin Sensitizers

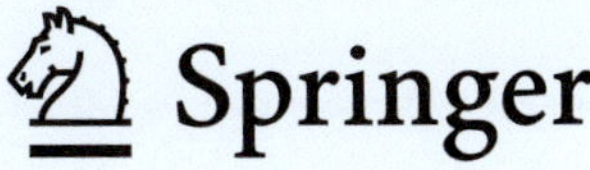 Springer

Mariagrazia Stracquadanio
Obstetrics and Gynecological Pathology
P.O. "S. Bambino", University of Catania
Catania
Italy

Lilliana Ciotta
Obstetric and Gynecological Pathology
P.O. "S. Bambino", University of Catania
Catania
Italy

ISBN 978-3-319-36668-5   ISBN 978-3-319-16760-2   (eBook)
DOI 10.1007/978-3-319-16760-2

Springer Cham Heidelberg New York Dordrecht London

Printed on acid-free paper

Springer International Publishing AG Switzerland is part of Springer Science+Business Media (www.springer.com)

Acknowledgments

A special thanks to "Oxford University" and "John Radcliffe Hospital – Cairns Library" for allowing the collection of the extended bibliography used.

Contents

1 Introduction 1
   1.1   PCOS Origins 1
   1.2   Definition and Epidemiology 2
   References 3

2 Etiopathogenesis 5
   2.1   Genetics of PCOS 5
   2.2   PCOS Physiopathology 10
   2.3   Role of Insulin in the Pathogenesis of PCOS 12
   References 15

3 Clinical Features 21
   3.1   Endocrine Aspects of PCOS 21
       3.1.1   Endocrine Pattern 21
       3.1.2   Clinical Endocrine Features 23
   3.2   Metabolic Aspects of PCOS 26
       3.2.1   The Role of the Adipocyte in Linking PCOS
               to Metabolic Syndrome 27
       3.2.2   The Role of Vitamin D in the Development
               of Metabolic Syndrome in PCOS Women 30
       3.2.3   Metabolic Syndrome and Associated Disorders 31
       3.2.4   Role of Insulin Resistance in Infertility
               and Pregnancy Outcome 39
   3.3   PCOS Phenotype in Different Ages 43
       3.3.1   Adolescence 43
       3.3.2   Fertile Period 45
       3.3.3   Premenopausal and Postmenopausal Period 45
   References 46

4 Psychological Implications of PCOS 63
   4.1   PCOS Symptoms and Psychological Correlation 63
       4.1.1   Obesity and Body Image 63
       4.1.2   Hirsutism 64
       4.1.3   Infertility and Sexual Life 64

   4.2   PCOS and Mental Disorders................................... 65
       4.2.1   Mood Disorders 65
       4.2.2   Anxiety... 66
       4.2.3   Eating Disorders................................. 67
   References 67

5 Diagnosis and Assessment...................................... 71
   5.1   Differential Diagnosis....................................... 71
   5.2   Risk Factors 72
   5.3   Clinical–Endocrine Features.................................. 72
       5.3.1   Oligomenorrhea and Anovulation 72
       5.3.2   Hirsutism 73
       5.3.3   Acne 73
   5.4   Endocrine Blood Tests 74
   5.5   Ultrasound Features 76
   5.6   Clinical–Metabolic Features.................................. 78
   5.7   Metabolic Blood Tests 81
       5.7.1   Glucose Metabolism Assessment and Calculation
            of Insulin Resistance 81
       5.7.2   Lipid and Hepatic Profile......................... 83
   References 84

6 PCOS Therapy... 89
   6.1   Diet and Exercise 89
       6.1.1   PCOS Dietary Recommendations 90
       6.1.2   Glycemic Index (GI) 92
       6.1.3   Glycemic Load (GL) 96
       6.1.4   Insulin Index.................................... 97
       6.1.5   Exercise 97
   6.2   Insulin-Sensitizing Agents and Statins......................... 98
       6.2.1   Thiazolidinediones.............................. 99
       6.2.2   Metformin...................................... 100
       6.2.3   Statins... 112
   6.3   Inositol and Other Supplements 113
       6.3.1   Inositol and Its Isomers 113
       6.3.2   Antioxidants.................................... 120
       6.3.3   Vitamin D...................................... 121
       6.3.4   Glucomannan 122
   References 122

Erratum E1

Introduction

1

1.1 PCOS Origins

Polycystic ovary syndrome (PCOS) is not a recent disorder, but it seems to be very old. Going back to the early history, Hippocrates and Soranus of Ephesus reported that "many women with masculine and robust aspect don't menstruate and they don't become pregnant" [1, 2].

Some authors suggest that the origin of PCOS began in Paleolithic communities, in which environmental stressful factors favored the survival of the "thrifty genotype": it was represented by males and females with the greatest capacity for energy storage necessary to face fasting periods [3, 4].

Moreover, subfertility among nomadic hunters gave some benefits: women could care only for one child, and a lower parity may have reduced the death rates of these women and the risk of progeny abandonment, as delivery-related complications were a major cause of mortality in reproductive-age women.

On the other hand, during the Neolithic revolution, when communities started to be sedentary, PCOS genotype may have survived because of its robustness, with some gene variants over the years, as well shown by the heterogeneity of PCOS phenotypes and genotypes.

Moreover, since the eighteenth century it was noticed that signs of hyperandrogenism were associated with metabolic abnormalities, such as increased visceral fat [5].

Jean Vague, physician and professor at University of Marseille, introduced the term "android obesity" to define the abdominal fat accumulation, which is the typical male pattern of body fat distribution, associated with increased diabetes and cardiovascular risk [6]. Later, it was realized that lots of hyperandrogenic women were obese with increased visceral fat; they had increased insulin response during OGTT (oral glucose tolerance test), and they presented with acanthosis nigricans [7, 8]: all of these are signs of insulin resistance, and these observations were the starting point for the study of the association between insulin resistance and PCOS.

© Springer International Publishing Switzerland 2015

M. Stracquadanio, L. Ciotta, *Metabolic Aspects of PCOS: Treatment with Insulin Sensitizers*, DOI 10.1007/978-3-319-16760-2_1

1.2   Definition and Epidemiology

Polycystic ovary syndrome (PCOS) is a heterogeneous endocrine and metabolic disorder, characterized by chronic anovulation/oligomenorrhea, hyperandrogenism, and insulin resistance.

In accordance with the most used guidelines drawn in Rotterdam in 2003 by ESHRE/ASRM (European Society for Human Reproduction and Embryology/American Society for Reproductive Medicine) [9], PCOS diagnosis can be raised only after the exclusion of other known causes of hyperandrogenism and amenorrhea (hyperprolactinemia, non-classic congenital adrenal 21-hydroxylase deficiency, thyroid dysfunction, androgen-secreting neoplasm, Cushing's syndrome) and when there are at least two of the three following parameters:

1. Oligomenorrhea or anovulatory cycles with menstrual irregularities
2. Elevated levels of circulating androgens or clinical manifestations of hyperandrogenism
3. Ultrasound evidence of micropolycystic ovaries

The previous criteria processed by NIH (National Institute of Health) in 1992 included both:

1. Clinical and/or biochemical hyperandrogenism
2. Menstrual dysfunction

The most recent (2006) AES (Androgen Excess Society) criteria [10] includes all of the following conditions:

1. Clinical and/or biochemical hyperandrogenism
2. Ovarian dysfunction and/or micropolycystic ovaries

Approximately 85–90 % of women with oligomenorrhea have PCOS, while 30–40 % of women with amenorrhea suffer from PCOS [11].

More than 80 % of women showing symptoms of androgen excess have PCOS [12]. Roughly 90–95 % of anovulatory women presenting to infertility clinics have PCOS. The syndrome is present in approximately 5–10 % of reproductive-age women, and it is considered the most frequent endocrine abnormality in females.

As there are significant variations in the clinical appearance of PCOS, its prevalence may be different among populations.

It is 4.8 and 8 % in white and black women in southeastern United States [13], 6.8 % in white women in Greece [14], 6.5 % in white women in Spain [15], 6.3 % in South Asian in Sri Lanka [16], and 5 % in Thai women [17].

Some groups have showed that the frequency of PCOS varies depending on the diagnostic criteria used: for example, the prevalence estimations using the Rotterdam criteria are two to three times greater than those achieved using NIH criteria [18–21].

For example, in China, Chen et al. reported that the prevalence in South Chinese population was 2.2 % based on NIH criteria [22], while in a cross-sectional epidemiologic investigation conducted in ten provinces of China, the prevalence of PCOS using the Rotterdam criteria was 5.61 % [23]. The difference may depend on the size of the sample and ethnicity too. The Rotterdam-PCOS group appeared to be more than 1.5–2 times larger than the group classified as NIH-PCOS [24].

References

1. Hanson AE (1975) Hippocrates: disease of women 1. Signs (Chic) 1:567–584
2. Temkin O (1991) Soranus' gynecology. The Johns Hopkins University Press, Baltimore
3. Chakravarthy MV, Booth FW (2004) Eating, exercise, and "thrifty" genotypes: connecting the dots toward an evolutionary understanding of modern chronic diseases. J Appl Physiol 96:3–10
4. Neel JV (1962) Diabetes mellitus: a "thrifty" genotype rendered detrimental by "progress"? Am J Hum Genet 14:353–362
5. Morgagni J (1765) De Sedibus et Causis Morborum per Anatomen Indagata (The seats and causes of diseases in- vestigated by anatomy), 2nd edn, Tomus primus. Sumptibus Remondinianis, Patavii
6. Vague J (1947) La differentiation sexuelle Facteur determinant des formes de l'obesite'. Presse Med 55:339–340
7. Dunaif A, Hoffman AR, Scully RE et al (1985) Clinical, biochemical, and ovarian morphologic features in women with acanthosis nigricans and masculinization. Obstet Gynecol 66:545–552
8. Flier JS, Eastman RC, Minaker KL et al (1985) Acanthosis nigricans in obese women with hyperandrogenism. Characterization of an insulin-resistant state distinct from the Type A and B syndromes. Diabetes 34:101–107
9. Rotterdam ESHRE/ASRM-Sponsored PCOS Consensus Workshop Group (2004) Revised (2003) consensus on diagnostic criteria and long- term health risks related to polycystic ovary syndrome. Fertil Steril 81:19–25
10. Azziz R, Carmina E, DeWailly D et al (2006) Position statement: criteria for defining polycystic ovary syndrome as a predominantly hyperandrogenic syndrome: an androgen excess society guideline. J Clin Endocrinol Metab 91:4237–4245
11. Hart R (2007) Definitions, prevalence and symptoms of polycystic ovaries and the polycystic ovary syndrome. In: Allahbadia GN, Agrawal R (eds) Polycystic ovary syndrome. Anshan, Ltd, Kent, pp 15–26
12. Azziz R, Sanchez L, Knochenhauer ES et al (2004) Androgen excess in women: experience with over 1,000 consecutive patients. J Clin Endocrinol Metab 89(2):453–462
13. Azziz R, Woods KS, Reyna R et al (2004) The prevalence and features of the polycystic ovary syndrome in an unselected population. J Clin Endocrinol Metab 89(6):2745–2749
14. Diamanti-Kandarakis E, Kouli CR, Bergiele AT et al (1999) A survey of the polycystic ovary syndrome in the Greek island of Lesbos: hormonal and metabolic profile. J Clin Endocrinol Metab 84(11):4006–4011
15. Asuncion M, Calvo RM, San MJ (2000) A prospective study of the prevalence of the polycystic ovary syndrome in unselected Caucasian women from Spain. J Clin Endocrinol Metab 85(7):2434–2438
16. Kumarapeli V, Seneviratne RA, Wijeyaratne CN et al (2008) A simple screening approach for assessing community prevalence and phenotype of polycystic ovary syndrome in a semi-urban population in Sri Lanka. Am J Epidemiol 168(3):321–328
17. Vutyavanich T, Khaniyao V, Wongtra-Ngan S (2007) Clinical, endocrine and ultrasonographic features of polycystic ovary syndrome in Thai women. J Obstet Gynaecol Res 33(5):677–680

18. March WA, Moore VM, Willson KJ et al (2010) The prevalence of polycystic ovary syndrome in a community sample assessed under contrasting diagnostic criteria. Hum Reprod 25(2):544–551
19. Mehrabian F, Khani B, Kelishadi R, Ghanbari E (2011) The prevalence of polycystic ovary syndrome in Iranian women based on different diagnostic criteria. Endokrynol Pol 62(3):238–242
20. Tehrani FR, Simbar M, Tohidi M et al (2011) The prevalence of polycystic ovary syndrome in a community sample of Iranian population: Iranian PCOS prevalence study. Reprod Biol Endocrinol 9:39
21. Yildiz BO, Bozdag G, Yapici Z et al (2012) Prevalence, phenotype and cardiometabolic risk of polycystic ovary syndrome under different diagnostic criteria. Hum Reprod 27(10): 3067–3073
22. Chen X, Yang D, Mo Y et al (2008) Prevalence of polycystic ovary syndrome in unselected women from southern China. Eur J Obstet Gynecol Reprod Biol 139(1):59–64
23. Zhao Y, Qiao J (2013) Ethnic differences in the phenotypic expression of polycystic ovary syndrome. Steroids 78:755–760
24. Broekmans FJ, Knauff EA, Valkenburg O et al (2006) PCOS according to the Rotterdam consensus criteria: change in prevalence among WHO-II anovulation and association with metabolic factors. BJOG 113(10):1210–1217

Etiopathogenesis

2

2.1 Genetics of PCOS

PCOS is a multifactorial polygenic disease (interaction between several genetic and environmental factors), with a heritability of $\sim$70 %. It is intrinsically difficult to study by a genetic point of view, and most of the current literature (>70 studies based on the candidate gene approach) is inconclusive, with many studies resulting inconsistent, controversial, and without a clear consensus [1].

In the first studies on the genetic basis of PCOS, both maternal and paternal patterns of inheritance are suggested: the incidence of oligomenorrhea and polycystic ovaries was found to be increased in first-degree relatives of PCOS patients compared with controls, and males in those families had increased hairiness according to the questionnaire, suggesting an autosomal dominant pattern of inheritance [2].

Recently, the inheritance was confirmed by some authors who found that PCOS was present in 35 % of the mothers and 40 % of the sisters of PCOS patients [3].

Moreover, increased incidence of insulin resistance in the fathers and brothers of PCOS women [4] has been considered as the "male phenotype" in PCOS families. The genes involved in the pathogenesis of hyperandrogenism are expressed in a variable way depending on the factors predominating in every different ethnic populations; this explains the phenotypic variability of hyperandrogenic disorders. Another theory is that the features of PCOS families result from nongenetic inheritance, and they are related to environmental factors that are present only in the affected families.

Ibanez hypothesized that some insults during pregnancy may induce to intrauterine growth retardation, which probably induces a "thrifty phenotype" in small for gestational age babies. These have a high risk of suffering from insulin resistance, which may result in hypertension, glucose intolerance, adrenal axis hyperactivity with relative cortisol excess, functional hyperandrogenism, and PCOS later in life, especially if they are exposed to environmental factors such as a sedentary lifestyle and a diet rich in saturated fat [5].

© Springer International Publishing Switzerland 2015
M. Stracquadanio, L. Ciotta, *Metabolic Aspects of PCOS: Treatment with Insulin Sensitizers*, DOI 10.1007/978-3-319-16760-2_2

These environmental factors may cluster in certain families because exercising and dieting are greatly influenced by parental lifestyle. The metabolic abnormalities of the "thrifty phenotype" can induce additional insult to the pregnancies of these SGA (small for gestational age) and PCOS women, and these defects might be transmitted to another generation without the participation of any genetic abnormality.

On the other hand, if small for gestational age babies have healthy habits, insulin resistance and its consequences might be improved, and theoretically, their fetuses will not be exposed to a hostile metabolic environment during pregnancy, preventing nongenetic inheritance of these conditions. However, intrauterine growth restriction might be influenced by genetic variants as well, and the most likely scenario is represented by an interaction between predisposing genetic abnormalities and unfavorable environmental conditions [6].

Thus, even if several studies conducted in families of women with PCOS have demonstrated the genetic basis of the syndrome, nowadays a genetic pattern certainly involved in PCOS predisposition has not been identified.

Most studies have included different kinds of genes: those related to androgen biosynthesis and action and their regulation, genes involved in insulin resistance and associated disorders, and also genes involved in chronic inflammation and atherosclerosis.

Among the genes involved in androgen biosynthesis, there are:

- *CYP17*: This gene encodes the P450c17α enzyme, which catalyzes the conversion of pregnenolone and progesterone into, respectively, 17-hydroxypregnenolone and 17-hydroxyprogesterone and of these steroids into dehydroepiandrosterone and androstenedione. In the past, the hyperactivity of this enzyme was correlated to hyperandrogenism [7].

  CYP17 is located in chromosome 10q24.3, and its promoter encloses a T/C SNP at 34 bp from the transcription start that might regulate enzyme activity. Some studies hypothesized that this polymorphism was associated with polycystic ovaries morphology on ultrasound [8, 9], and it was found that PCOS patients homozygous for C alleles of this polymorphism showed increased serum testosterone levels [10, 11].

  On the contrary, other studies suggested that this is a polymorphism without functional consequences for the development of polycystic ovaries and hyperandrogenism [12–14]. Besides, no significant evidence for linkage or association was found in a family-based genome study [15].

- *CYP11A*: This gene is located at 15q24 and encodes the cholesterol side chain cleavage enzyme, important for the conversion of cholesterol into progesterone, which is the first step in adrenal and ovarian steroidogenesis. A VNTR polymorphism, consisting in repeats of a (tttta)n pentanucleotide at −528 bp from the ATG start of translation site in the *CYP11A* promoter, might play a role in the pathogenesis of PCOS [16].

  Some studies confirmed its association with polycystic ovaries and hirsute women [16, 17], while other studies did not demonstrate linkage with the CYP11A locus in PCOS patients or association of CYP11A VNTR alleles with hyperandrogenism [18]. Moreover, recent experiments involving a large number of subjects concluded that the existence of associations between CYP11A promoter variation and androgen-related phenotypes had been considerably overestimated in previous studies [19].

- *CYP19*: This gene encodes aromatase, which converts androgens in estrogens. This enzyme maybe has a decreased activity in granulosa cells and follicles of PCOS women, and the consequent androgen excess might contribute to abnormal follicle development [20, 21]. On the contrary, no evidence for linkage of CYP19 with PCOS was found in other English and American studies [15, 16].
- *LH Gene*: LH hypersecretion is present in almost 50 % of PCOS women, and two mutations, Trp[8]Arg and Ile[15]Thr, could be the cause of an abnormal LH β molecule [22]. The first PCOS GWAS (genome-wide association studies) identified LH/choriogonadotropin receptor (LHCGR) as a susceptibility gene for PCOS: the interaction of LHCGR and its ligand, LH, plays a fundamental role in the folliculogenesis of mammals. A study suggested that LHCGR might participate in the physiopathology of PCOS by deviations in the methylation statuses of its promoter CpG sites, a hypomethylation in particular [23].
- *SHBG Genes*: Sex hormone-binding globulin (SHBG) controls the admission of testosterone and estradiol to target tissues.
  Decreased SHBG is an important feature of hyperandrogenic women, causing increased tissue androgen availability [24].
  Recently, an association between a (TAAAA)n polymorphism in the promoter of the SHBG gene and PCOS has been reported. Longer alleles (more than eight repeats) were frequent in Greek PCOS patients, while non-hyperandrogenic women presented with a higher frequency of shorter alleles [25].

The second group of genes includes those involved in insulin resistance and metabolic disorders, which are:

- *INSR* (*Insulin Receptor Gene*): Insulin resistance represents the major metabolic aspect of PCOS. INSR contains several polymorphisms, but most of them are silent or are located in intronic regions and are present with similar frequencies in patients with polycystic ovaries and hyperandrogenism and in controls [26]. Polymorphism in exon 17 of the tyrosine kinase domain is the only one found, but it was not associated to insulin resistance [27]. On the other hand, it was found that a C/T SNP at the tyrosine kinase domain of INSR is associated with PCOS, but further studies are needed to confirm it [6].
- *INS*: Pancreatic β-cell dysfunction in PCOS women seems to have a genetic origin as well. It was found that women with menstrual irregularities and/or hirsutism and polycystic ovaries, who were homozygous for class III alleles, were more frequently anovulatory and had increased BMI and fasting insulin compared with women homozygous for class I alleles. Paternal transmission of class III alleles from heterozygous fathers to anovulatory PCOS patients is more frequent than maternal transmission of the allele [28–30], and in addition, class III alleles predisposed these patients to both PCOS and type 2 diabetes mellitus.

However, other studies were not able to prove this [31, 32], and unluckily the INS locus was not associated with PCOS in an American linkage study on PCOS patients [15].

- *Insulin Growth Factor System Genes*: IGFs, their receptors, binding proteins, and proteases are important for the normal development of the ovary [33].
  They are peptide hormones secreted having important functions such as mediation of growth hormone action, stimulation of growth of cultured cells, stimulation of the action of insulin, and involvement in development and growth. IGFs stimulate ovarian cellular mitosis and steroidogenesis, inhibit apoptosis, and might be related to the development of functional hyperandrogenism and PCOS [34].
  In particular, IGF-2 stimulates adrenal and ovarian androgen secretion: the increased frequency of homozygosis for these alleles could contribute to hyperandrogenism in PCOS patients [35].
- *Peroxisome Proliferator-Activated Receptor-γ* (*PPAR-γ*): They are members of the nuclear receptor superfamily of ligand-activated transcription factors [36]. These genes are involved in adipocyte differentiation, lipid and glucose metabolism, and atherosclerosis [37]. The human PPAR-γ gene is composed of nine exons; recent studies have indicated that the modified Ala12 allele is involved in increased insulin sensitivity by enhanced suppression of lipid oxidation, enabling more efficient glucose disposal [38].
- *Calpain-10*: It is an enzyme that has an important role in insulin secretion and action [39]. The 112/121 haplotype combination of the University of Chicago single nucleotide polymorphisms (UCSNP)-43, UCSNP-19, and UCSNP-63 in the gene encoding calpain-10, located at 2q37.3, has been reported to increase the risk for diabetes [40]. Some authors found no association between this haplotype and PCOS patients [41, 42], while recently a Spanish study reported an association between PCOS and USCNP-44 [43, 44].

More recently, genes encoding inflammatory cytokines have been identified as target genes for PCOS, as pro-inflammatory genotypes and phenotypes are also associated with obesity, insulin resistance, type 2 diabetes, PCOS, and increased cardiovascular risk.

- *Paraoxonase* (*PON1*): The PON1 gene is mainly expressed in the liver and encodes for serum PON1, which is an antioxidant high-density lipoprotein-associated enzyme. Liver PON1 mRNA expression is influenced by genetic and environmental factors, and both androgens and pro-inflammatory mediators decrease liver PON1 expression [45].
  Homozygosis for T alleles of the −108C/T polymorphism in PON1 was more frequent in PCOS patients compared with non-hyperandrogenic women. Patients homozygous for −108T alleles of PON1 had increased hirsutism scores, total testosterone, and free testosterone and androstenedione levels related to those carriers of −108C alleles [35]. Nowadays, it is well known that oxidative stress

may damage insulin action. Indeed, reduced serum PON1 activity might contribute to the insulin resistance of PCOS patients [46].

- *TNF-α*: In vitro, this growth factor stimulates proliferation and steroidogenesis in theca cells and helps insulin and IGF-1 to exert their effects on the ovary [47]. Nine polymorphisms in the TNF-α gene were studied (−1196C/T, −1125G/C, −1031T/C, −863C/A, −857C/T, −316G/A, −308G/A, −238G/A, and −163G/A), but no differences between patients and controls were found: only lean hyperandrogenic patients showed increased serum TNF-α levels [48]. This finding might imply that TNF-α gene does not have a major role in PCOS etiology but could be a modifying factor for phenotypic features [6].
- *TNFR2 Gene (TNFRSF1B)*: TNFR2 mediates most of the metabolic effects of TNF-α [49]. The 196Arg allele of the $Met^{196}Arg$ (676T/G) polymorphism in exon 6 of this gene was more frequent in patients with PCOS compared with healthy controls, and it was hypothesized that it was responsible for modulating TNF-α in target tissues [50].
- *IL-6:* This cytokine seems to be implicated in insulin resistance mechanism, and increased levels were found in peritoneal fluid of anovulatory PCOS patients, suggesting a role in the pathogenesis of hyperandrogenic disorders [51]. Common polymorphisms in both subunits of the IL-6 receptor were studied, and the Arg148 allele of the $Gly^{148}Arg$ polymorphism in the gp130 gene was more frequent in controls compared with hyperandrogenic patients: control women had lower 11-deoxycortisol and 17-hydroxyprogesterone concentrations and a significant decrease in free testosterone levels, suggesting that this polymorphism might have a protective effect against androgen excess [52].

Moreover, there are also other genetic structural variations that regulate gene and phenotype expression, such as telomeres: they are at the ends of eukaryotic chromosomes and are specialized chromatin structures composed of highly conserved tandem hexameric nucleotide repeats—TTAGGG—that extend for several kilobases [53]. Telomeres shorten progressively with each cell division, and their length is largely inherited and modulated by a variety of genetic and environmental factors [54]. Short telomeres can cause chromosomal instability, and this could be the reason of genetic mutations and chromosome abnormalities.

There is a correlation between oxidative stress and PCOS and between oxidative stress and telomere length. For this reason, it has been hypothesized that telomere length plays an important role in the pathophysiology of PCOS.

In a Chinese study, the mean telomere length was measured in a large cohort of PCOS patients and controls, and the association between telomere length and this endocrine–metabolic disease was analyzed. A significant reduction of telomere length was observed in PCOS patients compared with healthy controls. Individuals with the shorter telomere length had significantly higher disease risk than those with the longest telomere length, after adjustment for age. One possible mechanism for the shortened telomeres in PCOS patients is that some etiological factors of PCOS, such as androgen excess, abdominal adiposity, insulin resistance, and obesity, could contribute to raised oxidative stress that leads to telomere shortening. This could represent a negative feedback cycle in which shortened telomeres, in turn, affect endocrine-, metabolic-, or reproductive-related gene expression and worsen the abnormal metabolic phenotypes of the disease [55].

2.2   PCOS Physiopathology

It has been shown that polycystic ovary presents a greater number of small antral follicles (2–9 mm in diameter) than the normal ovary. This morphological scenario could be the consequence of a potential dysregulation of the recruitment mechanism of primordial follicles that, on the contrary, are present in physiological number.

On the other hand, the final pathway of follicular growth, which is gonadotropin dependent, is blocked in the majority of PCOS patients, and it is the basis of anovulation and oligo-/amenorrhea.

In a normal cycle, only the dominant follicle responds to LH action when it reaches 10 mm in diameter. In PCOS patients, the response to LH occurs inappropriately in smaller follicles; a large number of antral follicles reach a terminal differentiation before the appropriate time, producing a larger amount of steroids and inhibin B that have a negative feedback on the production of FSH: the result is the arrest of follicular growth.

As underlined before, the etiology of this syndrome is still partly unknown, but it is likely to be multifactorial. The most significant theories are explained below:

- *Exaggerated Adrenarche*: It is possible that PCOS might be established and maintained in response to an abnormal adrenal hypersecretion of androgens due to congenital adrenal enzyme deficiency [56].

  Yen suggested an etiopathogenetic model, which provides, in response to a stress condition, a transient adrenal androgen hypersecretion, triggering an abnormal pattern of the pituitary gonadotropins' pulsatility. As puberty progresses, the adrenal cortex is replaced by ovaries in maintaining the hypersecretion of androgens.

  Finally, the increase in ovarian androgen level changes adrenal specific enzyme activities involved in the process of steroidogenesis [57].

- *Abnormal Secretion of Gonadotropins*: The high levels of LH in women with PCOS are due to greater amplitude of the peaks of this hormone and its increased frequency of pulsatility; on the contrary, the average concentration of FSH is mostly decreased. The high levels of LH are not caused by an inability of the hypothalamic-pituitary axis to respond to the negative feedback exerted by estrogen, but it might be caused by the high pituitary sensitivity to LH-RH. The chronically elevated and acyclic levels of estrogens in PCOS patients may, in turn, increase both the basal levels of LH and LH response to GnRH.

  Moreover, an elevated endogenous opioid tone might cause an exceeding GnRH release with a following abnormal LH pulsatility, causing increased level of LH-dependent ovarian androgens [58].

- *Rosenfield's Hypothesis*: Rosenfield suggested that PCOS results from a hyper-activity of cytochrome P450c17α in the ovarian theca cells. This enzymatic complex binds progesterone and converts it sequentially in 17-hydroxyproges-terone (via a 17α-hydroxylation) and androstenedione (via a C-17,20-lytic activity). The steroidogenetic route particularly involved in the ovary is the Δ-4 pathway.

  Moreover, at adrenal level, cytochrome P450c17α forms 17-ketosteroids, espe-cially using the Δ-5 steroidogenetic pathway, and it creates more dehydroepian-drosterone than androstenedione. An abnormal regulation of this enzyme activity, therefore, both at ovarian and adrenal levels, could explain the androgenic hyper-function of both glands, as occurs in PCOS.

  Rosenfield proposed three hypotheses to explain the hyperactivity of this enzy-matic complex:

  1. The hyperactivity is the result of an increased LH release, characteristic of PCOS.
  2. The action of LH on theca cells is increased and amplified, even in the pres-ence of normal levels of LH.
  3. In PCOS women, ovarian theca cells might work in a way more similar to the testicular Leydig cells rather than those of the normal ovarian theca cells, because in the ovarian stroma, some "aberrant" cells (called "lipid cell rest") in which an abnormal steroidogenic secretory pattern is established, could exist.

  However, according to Rosenfield, the hyperactivity of cytochrome P45017α cannot be the unique cause of PCOS, but it is part of a more complex etiopatho-genetic model [59].

- *Hyperestronemia*: Increased levels of estrone (E_1), characteristic of polycystic ovary, are able to modify the normal patterns of gonadotropins' pulsatility. This high E_1 level in PCOS women is generally the result of an increased ovarian production of androstenedione (A) and its conversion into E_1 by a specific FSH-dependent enzyme called aromatase.

  This enzyme is present in adipose tissue; thus, overweight or obese women have a greater amount of enzyme and, consequently, more estrone compared to normal-weight subjects. Alternatively, estrone levels might be increased in lean women with high production of androstenedione. The part of testosterone con-verted to estrone is very poor, and probably for this reason, the hypertestostero-nemia per se is not able to affect significantly the gonadotropins' pulsatility [60]. Many women with PCOS are overweight or obese: these conditions are usually associated with low levels of SHBG. This globulin binds both testosterone and estradiol: thus, in conditions in which SHBG is reduced, consequently, estradiol free fraction (the most biologically active) is increased.

  This condition causes a negative impact on the release of FSH with consequent alteration of folliculogenesis process and increased release of LH, which is fol-lowed by an increased ovarian androgen synthesis.

  In addition, the increase of androgen plasma levels contributes to the reduction of hepatic biosynthesis of SHBG.

• *Hyperinsulinemia*: High level of insulin accelerates the development of granulosa cell LH responsiveness by amplifying the induction of LH receptors, and thus, it induces a block of follicular growth with multiple small follicle formation.

The role of insulin is properly discussed in Sect. 2.3.

2.3   Role of Insulin in the Pathogenesis of PCOS

Insulin controls glucose homeostasis stimulating glucose uptake by tissues that are responsive to insulin (adipocytes, skeletal and cardiac muscle) and by suppressing hepatic glucose production [61, 62]. In addition, insulin decreases free fatty acid levels by suppressing lipolysis [63], and it promotes cell growth and differentiation [64].

"Insulin resistance" is defined as "a decreased ability of insulin to mediate its metabolic actions on glucose uptake, glucose production and lipolysis, requiring increased amounts of insulin to achieve its proper metabolic action."

In fact, increased circulating insulin levels characterize insulin resistance if pancreatic β-cells are functionally intact [65].

Insulin exerts its function by binding to its cell surface receptor; ligand binding induces auto-phosphorylation of the insulin receptor on specific tyrosine residues, and this actives its intrinsic kinase activity, while serine phosphorylation inhibits it [66, 67].

The tyrosine-phosphorylated insulin receptor phosphorylates, in turn, intracellular substrates, such as IRS 1–4, Shc, and APS to start signal transduction [68–70].

Insulin stimulates glucose uptake by translocating GLUT-4 (the insulin-responsive glucose transporter) from intracellular vesicles to the cell surface [68, 70].

This pathway is mediated by activation of PI3K and Akt/PKB, which also leads to serine phosphorylation of GSK3 (glycogen synthase kinase 3), resulting in inhibition of its kinase activity: this inhibition causes dephosphorylation of glycogen synthase, increasing glycogen synthesis, and also dephosphorylation of eIF2B which increase protein synthesis [64, 70].

Insulin has also an important mitogenic action: it stimulates cell growth and differentiation through the MAPK-ERK pathway [64].

This route is activated by insulin receptor-mediated phosphorylation of Shc or IRS, which stimulates a cascade of serine/threonine kinase resulting in stimulation of MAP kinase and MAPK-ERK 1/2. ERK 1/2 translocates to the nucleus and phosphorylates transcription factors to start cell growth and differentiation.

This mitogenic pathway can be altered without affecting the metabolic actions of insulin and vice versa [64].

Insulin signaling can be terminated by dephosphorylation of the receptor by tyrosine phosphatases; in addition, serine phosphorylation (mediated by serine kinases) of the insulin receptor and its substrates can decrease insulin signaling as well [64, 70].

There is a post-binding defect in insulin signaling in PCOS women, resulting in marked insulin sensitivity decrease. The defect is due to serine phosphorylation of the insulin receptor and IRS-1 secondary to intracellular serine kinases. This causes a decreased activation of PI3K mediated by insulin and resistance to the metabolic actions of insulin too [71].

Moreover, supporting this theory, it was shown that serine kinase inhibitors corrected the phosphorylation defect, underlining the role of a serine kinase extrinsic to the insulin receptor as the cause of decreased receptor auto-phosphorylation. This defect in the first phases of the insulin signaling pathway is present in adipocytes [72, 73] and skeletal muscle [71, 74], which are the most important target tissues for glucose uptake stimulated by insulin.

Even if obesity is the major contributing factor for insulin resistance in PCOS women, dysfunction in post-receptor mechanism action could be a good explanation for insulin-resistant lean/normal-weight PCOS women.

Moreover, ovarian granulosa lutein cells could be considered a selective target tissue too, in which insulin resistance is selective, affecting only the metabolic but not the mitogenic action of insulin.

In addition, it has been taken into consideration the crucial role of serum fetuin-α in the inhibition of insulin receptor tyrosine kinase activity [75].

It is a carrier protein like albumin, and a recent study has shown that fetuin-α serum levels are higher in PCOS women, having probably a role in triggering the processes that lead to insulin resistance and androgen excess in PCOS [76].

Furthermore, it was supposed that hyperinsulinemia might be the result of a decreased insulin clearance or of an increased insulin secretion [77, 78].

Insulin clearance is receptor mediated; thus, insulin-resistant patients are supposed to have a decreased clearance because of intrinsic or acquired decrease in receptor number and/or function [78, 79].

Some authors have shown that fasting hyperinsulinemia in PCOS women is the result of a combination of increased basal insulin secretion and decreased hepatic insulin clearance [80, 81].

Lots of evidence demonstrate a direct insulin action on ovarian steroidogenesis and the importance of the insulin signaling pathway in the control of ovulation. Obviously, insulin receptors are present both in normal and polycystic ovary syndrome women. IGF-1 (insulin growth factor 1) is synthetized by the ovary, and its receptor is a tyrosine kinase with few structural and functional homologies with the insulin receptor [82, 83].

Insulin can bind to the IGF-1 receptor activating it, and IGF-1 can bind to and activate the insulin receptor [84, 85].

The affinity of the IGF-1 receptor for insulin is less than it is for IGF-1 and vice versa; despite this, the two receptors can assemble together to form a hybrid tetramer, which is able to bind insulin and IGF-1 in the same way. Therefore, some insulin action on the ovary may be mediated by IGF-1 or hybrid insulin–IGF-1 receptor [86, 87].

Some studies have shown that insulin action on steroidogenesis in granulosa and theca cells is mediated via insulin receptor, both in normal and PCOS women [88, 89]. Moreover, in PCOS granulosa cells, increased insulin levels might cause premature LH receptor expression in small follicles, leading to premature granulosa terminal differentiation and the arrest of follicular growth, which is the basis for anovulation.

In normal theca cells, insulin and LH activate 17α-hydroxylase activity of P450c17α, a crucial enzyme in the regulation of androgen biosynthesis encoded by CYP17, via PI3K signaling; inhibition of MAPK-ERK1/2 signaling has no effect on 17α-hydroxylase activity [89].

It seems that PCOS theca cells are more responsive to the androgen-stimulating insulin actions rather than normal controls [90].

Physiologically, insulin acts as a "co-gonadotropin" to increase androgen synthesis induced by LH in theca cells [91–93] and to boost FSH-mediated estrogen production and LH-induced luteinization in granulosa cells [94].

Furthermore, human studies have demonstrated that insulin can increase circulating androgen levels in PCOS women: insulin infusion during euglycemic clamp studies increased androgen level without altering gonadotropin secretion, suggesting a direct effect on steroidogenesis [95, 96].

Suppressing insulin levels leads to decreased testosterone levels in women with PCOS, while there is an increase in SHBG levels [97–99]. Thus, low insulinemia is the basis for normal to low androgen production in the ovary and for increasing SHBG levels which leads to low circulating active androgen levels too.

The correlation between PCOS, insulin, hyperandrogenism, and ovarian dysfunction is well exemplified in Fig. 2.1.

Moreover, insulin action on adrenal androgen production and gonadotropin secretion is not yet well known. Lowering insulin levels with ISD (insulin-sensitizing drugs) resulted in DHEAS decrease in PCOS women [100, 101]; other studies also suggested that insulin resistance and consequent hyperinsulinemia cause a reduced pituitary sensitivity to GnRH, contributing to anovulatory syndrome [102, 103].

According to all these findings, insulin could be defined as a "reproductive hormone" as well.

The central paradox in the pathophysiologic association between hyperinsulinemia and hyperandrogenemia in PCOS is that the ovary remains sensitive to insulin activity and consequent androgen production, despite a systemic insulin resistance: it is the so-called *selective insulin resistance* theory [104].

On the other hand, androgens can produce insulin resistance by direct effects on the skeletal muscle and adipose tissue insulin action, by altering adipokine secretion, and by increasing visceral adiposity, even if these effects on insulin actions are modest [105].

Additionally, adipose tissue in PCOS women is characterized by hypertrophic adipocytes and impaired lipolysis and insulin action. TNF-α, as well as other adipokines involved in insulin resistance, is altered in these kinds of patients [106].

Adiponectin applies insulin-sensitizing properties by stimulating fatty acid oxidation and reducing hepatic gluconeogenesis: some studies hypothesized that its dysregulation could be implicated in the pathogenesis of insulin resistance [107].

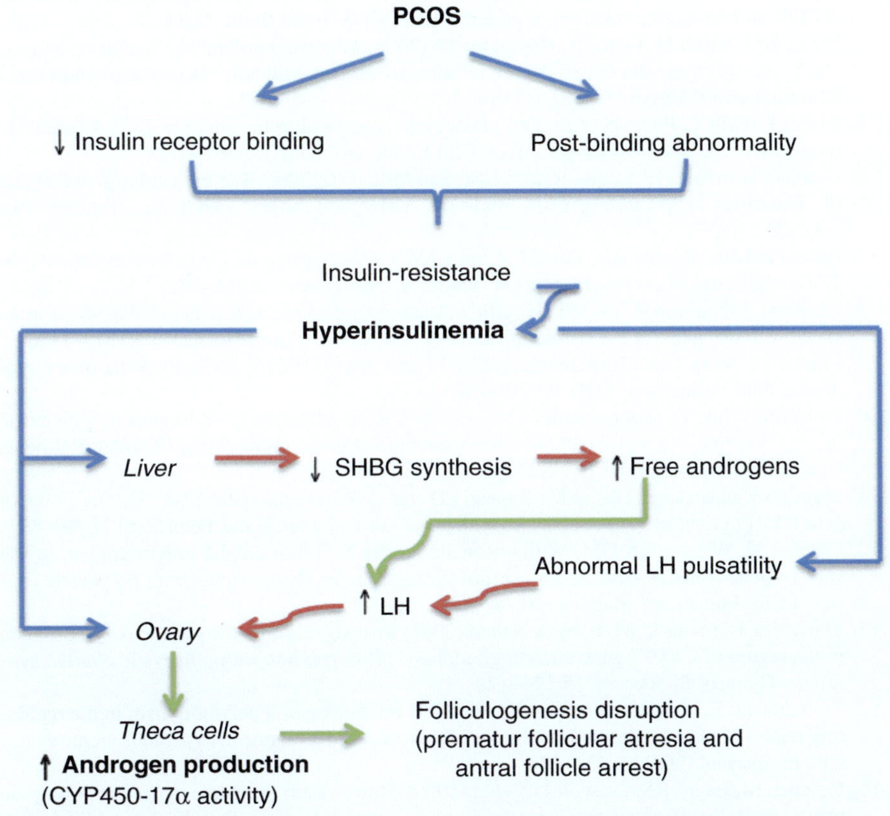

Fig. 2.1 Correlation between PCOS, hyperinsulinemia, hyperandrogenism, and ovarian dysfunction

TNF-α is secreted by adipose tissue macrophages and has pro-inflammatory properties: it causes serine phosphorylation of the insulin receptor substrate (IRS-1).

IGFBP3 is secreted by hepatic Kupffer cells and inhibits insulin-stimulated glucose uptake by dephosphorylating insulin receptor.

Both TNF-α and IGFBP3 might inhibit transcription of adiponectin, contributing to insulin resistance [108]: in fact low levels of adiponectin were found in patients with PCOS [109].

References

1. Barber TM, Franks S (2013) Genetics of polycystic ovary syndrome. Front Horm Res 40:28–39
2. Cooper HE, Spellacy WN, Prem KA, Cohen WD (1968) Hereditary factors in the Stein-Leventhal syndrome. Am J Obstet Gynecol 100:371–387

3. Kahsar-Miller MD, Nixon C, Boots LR et al (2001) Prevalence of polycystic ovary syndrome (PCOS) in first-degree relatives of patients with PCOS. Fertil Steril 75:53–58
4. Yildiz BO, Yarali H, Oguz H, Bayraktar M (2003) Glucose intolerance, insulin resistance, and hyperandrogenemia in first degree relatives of women with polycystic ovary syndrome. J Clin Endocrinol Metab 88:2031–2036
5. Ibanez L, Valls C, Potau N et al (2001) Polycystic ovary syndrome after precocious pubarche: ontogeny of the low-birthweight effect. Clin Endocrinol (Oxf) 55:667–672
6. Escobar-Morreale HF, Luque-Ramirez M, San Millan JL (2005) The molecular-genetic basis of functional hyperandrogenism and the polycystic ovary syndrome. Endocr Rev 26(2):251–282
7. Rosenfield RL, Barnes RB, Cara JF, Lucky AW (1990) Dysregulation of cytochrome P450c 17α as the cause of polycystic ovarian syndrome. Fertil Steril 53:785–791
8. Franks S, Williamson R (1994) Polycystic ovaries and premature male pattern baldness are associated with one allele of the steroid metabolism gene CYP17. Hum Mol Genet 3:1873–1876
9. Franks S (1997) The 17-hydroxylase/17,20 lyase gene (CYP17) and polycystic ovary syndrome. Clin Endocrinol (Oxf) 46:135–136
10. Franks S, White D, Gilling-Smith C et al (1996) Hypersecretion of androgens by polycystic ovaries: the role of genetic factors in the regulation of cytochrome P450c17 alpha. Baillieres Clin Endocrinol Metab 10:193–203
11. Diamanti-Kandarakis E, Bartzis MI, Zapanti ED et al (1999) Polymorphism T–C SNP (at 34 bp) of gene CYP17 promoter in Greek patients with polycystic ovary syndrome. Fertil Steril 71:431–435
12. Gharani N, Waterworth DM, Williamson R, Franks S (1996) 5alpha polymorphism of the CYP17 gene is not associated with serum testosterone levels in women with polycystic ovaries. J Clin Endocrinol Metab 81:4174
13. Marszalek B, Lacinski M, Babych N et al (2001) Investigations on the genetic polymorphism in the region of CYP17 gene encoding 5alpha-UTR in patients with polycystic ovarian syndrome. Gynecol Endocrinol 15:123–128
14. Techatraisak K, Conway GS, Rumsby G (1997) Frequency of a polymorphism in the regulatory region of the 17alpha-hydroxylase-17,20-lyase (CYP17) gene in hyperandrogenic states. Clin Endocrinol (Oxf) 46:131–134
15. Urbanek M, Legro RS, Driscoll DA et al (1999) Thirty-seven candidate genes for polycystic ovary syndrome: strongest evidence for linkage is with follistatin. Proc Natl Acad Sci U S A 96:8573–8578
16. Gharani N, Waterworth DM, Batty S et al (1997) Association of the steroid synthesis gene CYP11a with polycystic ovary syndrome and hyperandrogenism. Hum Mol Genet 6:397–402
17. Diamanti-Kandarakis E, Bartzis MI, Bergiele AT et al (2000) Microsatellite polymorphism (tttta) at -528 base pairs of gene CYP11a influences hyperandrogenemia in patients with polycystic ovary syndrome. Fertil Steril 73:735–741
18. San Millan JL, Sancho J, Calvo RM, Escobar-Morreale HF (2001) Role of the pentanucleotide (tttta)(n) polymorphism in the promoter of the CYP11a gene in the pathogenesis of hirsutism. Fertil Steril 75:797–802
19. Gaasenbeek M, Powell BL, Sovio U et al (2004) Large-scale analysis of the relationship between CYP11A promoter variation, polycystic ovarian syndrome, and serum testosterone. J Clin Endocrinol Metab 89:2408–2413
20. Takayama K, Fukaya T, Sasano H et al (1996) Immunohistochemical study of steroidogenesis and cell proliferation in polycystic ovarian syndrome. Hum Reprod 11:1387–1392
21. Jakimiuk AJ, Weitsman SR, Brzechffa PR, Magoffin DA (1998) Aromatase mRNA expression in individual follicles from polycystic ovaries. Mol Hum Reprod 4:1–8
22. Furui K, Suganuma N, Tsukahara S et al (1994) Identification of two point mutations in the gene coding luteinizing hormone (LH) β-subunit, associated with immunologically anomalous LH variants. J Clin Endocrinol Metab 78:107–113
23. Wang P et al (2014) Hypomethylation of the LH/choriogonadotropin receptor promoter region is a potential mechanism underlying susceptibility to polycystic ovary syndrome. Endocrinology 155(4):1445–1452

24. Pugeat M, Crave JC, Tourniaire J, Forest MG (1996) Clinical utility of sex hormone-binding globulin measurement. Horm Res 45:148–155
25. Xita N, Tsatsoulis A, Chatzikyriakidou A, Georgiou I (2003) Association of the (TAAAA)n repeat polymorphism in the sex hormone-binding globulin (SHBG) gene with polycystic ovary syndrome and relation to SHBG serum levels. J Clin Endocrinol Metab 88:5976–5980
26. Talbot JA, Bicknell EJ, Rajkhowa M et al (1996) Molecular scanning of the insulin receptor gene in women with polycystic ovarian syndrome. J Clin Endocrinol Metab 81:1979–1983
27. Conway GS, Avey C, Rumsby G (1994) The tyrosine kinase domain of the insulin receptor gene is normal in women with hyperinsulinaemia and polycystic ovary syndrome. Hum Reprod 9:1681–1683
28. Waterworth DM, Bennett ST, Gharani N et al (1997) Linkage and association of insulin gene VNTR regulatory polymorphism with polycystic ovary syndrome. Lancet 349:986–990
29. Michelmore K, Ong K, Mason S et al (2001) Clinical features in women with polycystic ovaries: relationships to insulin sensitivity, insulin gene VNTR and birth weight. Clin Endocrinol (Oxf) 55:439–446
30. Eaves IA, Bennett ST, Forster P et al (1999) Transmission ratio distortion at the INS-IGF2 VNTR. Nat Genet 22:324–325
31. Calvo RM, Telleria D, Sancho J et al (2002) Insulin gene variable number of tandem repeats regulatory polymorphism is not associated with hyperandrogenism in Spanish women. Fertil Steril 77:666–668
32. Vankova M, Vrbikova J, Hill M et al (2002) Association of insulin gene VNTR polymorphism with polycystic ovary syndrome. Ann NY Acad Sci 967:558–565
33. Voutilainen R, Franks S, Mason HD, Martikainen H (1996) Expression of insulin-like growth factor (IGF), IGF-binding protein, and IGF receptor messenger ribonucleic acids in normal and polycystic ovaries. J Clin Endocrinol Metab 81:1003–1008
34. Giudice LC (1999) Growth factor action on ovarian function in polycystic ovary syndrome. Endocrinol Metab Clin N Am 28:325–339
35. San Millan JL, Corton M, Villuendas G et al (2004) Association of the polycystic ovary syndrome with genomic variants related to insulin resistance, type 2 diabetes mellitus, and obesity. J Clin Endocrinol Metab 89:2640–2646
36. Issemann I, Green S (1990) Activation of a member of the steroid hormone receptor superfamily by peroxisome proliferators. Nature 347(6294):645–650
37. Li AC, Glass CK (2004) PPAR- and LXR-dependent pathways controlling lipid metabolism and the development of atherosclerosis. J Lipid Res 45(12):2161–2173
38. Lakkakula B, Thangavelu M, Godla U (2013) Genetic variants associated with insulin signaling and glucose homeostasis in the pathogenesis of insulin resistance in polycystic ovary syndrome: a systematic review. J Assist Reprod Genet 30:883–895
39. Sreenan SK, Zhou YP, Otani K et al (2001) Calpains play a role in insulin secretion and action. Diabetes 50:2013–2020
40. Horikawa Y, Oda N, Cox NJ et al (2000) Genetic variation in the gene encoding calpain-10 is associated with type 2 diabetes mellitus. Nat Genet 26:163–175
41. Ehrmann DA, Schwarz PE, Hara M et al (2002) Relationship of calpain-10 genotype to phenotypic features of polycystic ovary syndrome. J Clin Endocrinol Metab 87:1669–1673
42. Haddad L, Evans JC, Gharani N et al (2002) Variation within the type 2 diabetes susceptibility gene calpain-10 and polycystic ovary syndrome. J Clin Endocrinol Metab 87:2606–2610
43. Gonzalez A, Abril E, Roca A et al (2002) CAPN10 alleles are associated with polycystic ovary syndrome. J Clin Endocrinol Metab 87:3971–3976
44. Gonzalez A, Abril E, Roca A et al (2003) Specific CAPN10 gene haplotypes influence the clinical profile of polycystic ovary patients. J Clin Endocrinol Metab 88:5529–5536
45. Bin Ali A, Zhang Q, Lim YK et al (2003) Expression of major HDL-associated antioxidant PON-1 is gender dependent and regulated during inflammation. Free Radic Biol Med 34:824–829
46. Rudich A, Kozlovsky N, Potashnik R, Bashan N (1997) Oxidant stress reduces insulin responsiveness in 3T3–L1 adipocytes. Am J Physiol 272:E935–E940

47. Spaczynski RZ, Arici A, Duleba AJ (1999) Tumor necrosis factor-α stimulates proliferation of rat ovarian theca-interstitial cells. Biol Reprod 61:993–998
48. Escobar-Morreale HF, Calvo RM, Sancho J, San Millan JL (2001) TNF-α and hyperandrogenism: a clinical, biochemical, and molecular genetic study. J Clin Endocrinol Metab 86:3761–3767
49. Bazzoni F, Beutler B (1996) The tumor necrosis factor ligand and receptor families. N Engl J Med 334:1717–1725
50. Peral B, San Millan JL, Castello R et al (2002) The methionine 196 arginine polymorphism in exon 6 of the TNF receptor 2 gene (TNFRSF1B) is associated with the polycystic ovary syndrome and hyperandrogenism. J Clin Endocrinol Metab 87:3977–3983
51. Omu AE, Al-Azemi MK, Makhseed M et al (2003) Differential expression of T-helper cytokines in the peritoneal fluid of women with normal ovarian cycle compared with women with chronic anovulation. Acta Obstet Gynecol Scand 82:603–609
52. Escobar-Morreale HF, Calvo RM, Villuendas G et al (2003) Association of polymorphisms in the interleukin 6 receptor complex with obesity and hyperandrogenism. Obes Res 11:987–996
53. Blackburn EH (2001) Switching and signaling at the telomere. Cell 106:661–673
54. Nordfjäll K, Larefalk A, Lindgren P et al (2005) Telomere length and heredity: indications of paternal inheritance. Proc Natl Acad Sci U S A 102:16374–16378
55. Li Q et al (2014) A possible new mechanism in the pathophysiology of polycystic ovary syndrome (PCOS): the discovery that leukocyte telomere length is strongly associated with PCOS. J Clin Endocrinol Metab 99(2):E234–E240
56. Topolino A, Nappi C (1995) PCOS and adrenal function. In: Genazzani, Petraglia, Facchinetti: Atti del 4th world congress of gynecological endocrinology. Madonna di Campiglio, Parthenon
57. Ciotta L, Carcò C, Di Grazia S, Palumbo G (1996) La sindrome dell'ovaio policistico: profilo etiopatogenetico, problematiche diagnostiche e terapeutiche. Riv Ost Gin 1:67
58. Udolff L, Adashi EY (1995) Polycystic ovarian disease: a new look at an old subject. Curr Opin Obstet Gynecol 7:340
59. Ehrman D, Barnes R, Rosenfield RL (1995) Polycystic ovary syndrome as a form of functional ovarian hyperandrogenism due to dysregulation of androgen secretion. Endocr Rev 16(3): 322–353
60. Gonzalez F, Speroff L (1990) Adrenal morphologic consideration in polycystic ovary syndrome. Obstet Gynecol Surv 45(8):491–508
61. De Fronzo RA (1988) Lilly lecture (1987). The triumvirate: β-cell, muscle, liver. A collusion responsible for NIDDM. Diabetes 37(667–687):161
62. Bergman RN (2007) Orchestration of glucose homeostasis: from a small acorn to the California oak. Diabetes 56(1489–1501):162
63. Groop LC, Bonadonna RC, Simonson DC et al (1992) Effect of insulin on oxidative and non oxidative pathways of free fatty acid metabolism in human obesity. Am J Physiol 263:E79–E84
64. Saltiel AR, Kahn CR (2001) Insulin signaling and the regulation of glucose and lipid metabolism. Nature 414:799–806
65. Kahn CR (1985) The molecular mechanism of insulin action. Ann Rev Med 36:429–451
66. Kasuga M, Zick Y, Blith DL et al (1982) Insulin stimulation of phosphorylation of the subunit of the insulin receptor. Formation of both phosphoserine and phosphotyrosine. J Biol Chem 257(244):9891–9894
67. Shoelson SE, Boni-Schnetzler M, Pilch PF, Kahn CR (1991) Autophosphorylation within insulin receptor α-subunits can occur as an intramolecular process. Biochemistry 30:7740–7746
68. Cheatham B, Kahn CR (1995) Insulin action and the insulin signaling network. Endocr Rev 16:117–142
69. Myers MG Jr, Sun XJ, White MF (1994) The IRS-1 signaling system. Trends Biochem Sci 19:289–293
70. Choi K, Kim YB (2010) Molecular mechanism of insulin resistance in obesity and type 2 diabetes. Korean J Intern Med 25:119–129

71. Dunaif A, Xia J, Book CB et al (1995) Excessive insulin receptor serine phosphorylation in cultured fibroblasts and in skeletal muscle. J Clin Invest 96:801–810
72. Dunaif A, Segal KR, Shelley DR et al (1992) Evidence for distinctive and intrinsic defects in insulin action in polycystic ovary syndrome. Diabetes 41:1257–1266
73. Ciaraldi TP, el-Roeiy A, Madar Z et al (1992) Cellular mechanisms of insulin resistance in polycystic ovarian syndrome. J Clin Endocrinol Metab 75:577–583
74. Dunaif A, Wu X, Lee A, Diamanti-Kandarakis E (2001) Defects in insulin receptor signaling in vivo in the polycystic ovary syndrome (PCOS). Am J Physiol Endocrinol Metab 281:E392–E399
75. Mathews ST, Chellam N, Srinivas PR et al (2000) Alpha2-HSG, a specific inhibitor of insulin receptor autophosphorylation, interacts with the insulin receptor. Mol Cell Endocrinol 164:87–98
76. Enli Y et al (2013) Serum fetuin-A levels, insulin resistance and oxidative stress in women with polycystic ovary syndrome. Gynecol Endocrinol 29(12):1036–1039
77. Hucking K, Watanabe RM, Stefanovski D, Bergman RN (2008) OGTT-derived measures of insulin sensitivity are confounded by factors other than insulin sensitivity itself. Obesity (Silver Spring) 16:1938–1945
78. Flier JS, Minaker KL, Landsberg L et al (1982) Impaired in vivo insulin clearance in patients with severe target-cell resistance to insulin. Diabetes 31:132–135
79. Marshall S (1985) Kinetics of insulin receptor internalization and recycling in adipocytes. Shunting of receptors to a degradative pathway by inhibitors of recycling. J Biol Chem 260:4136–4144
80. O'Meara NM, Blackman JD, Ehrmann DA et al (1993) Defects in β-cell function in functional ovarian hyperandrogenism. J Clin Endocrinol Metab 76:1241–1247
81. Peiris AN, Mueller RA, Struve MF et al (1987) Relationship of androgenic activity to splanchnic insulin metabolism and peripheral glucose utilization in premenopausal women. J Clin Endocrinol Metab 64:162–169
82. El-Roeiy A, Chen X, Roberts VJ et al (1993) Expression of insulin-like growth factor-I (IGF-I) and IGF-II and the IGF-I, IGF-II, and insulin receptor genes and localization of the gene products in the human ovary. J Clin Endocrinol Metab 77:1411–1418
83. El-Roeiy A, Chen X, Roberts VJ et al (1994) Expression of the genes encoding the insulin-like growth factors (IGF-I and II), the IGF and insulin receptors, and IGF-binding proteins-1–6 and the localization of their gene products in normal and polycystic ovary syndrome ovaries. J Clin Endocrinol Metab 78:1488–1496
84. Czech MP (1982) Structural and functional homologies in the receptors for insulin and the insulin-like growth factors. Cell 31:8–10
85. Froesch ER, Zapf J (1985) Insulin-like growth factors and insulin: comparative aspects. Diabetologia 28:485–493
86. LeRoith D, Werner H, Beitner-Johnson D, Roberts CT Jr (1995) Molecular and cellular aspects of the insulin-like growth factor I receptor. Endocr Rev 16:143–163
87. Poretsky L (1991) On the paradox of insulin-induced hyperandrogenism in insulin-resistant states. Endocr Rev 12:3–13
88. Willis D, Franks S (1995) Insulin action in human granulosa cells from normal and polycystic ovaries is mediated by the insulin receptor and not the type-I insulin-like growth factor receptor. J Clin Endocrinol Metab 80:3788–3790
89. Munir I, Yen HW, Geller DH et al (2004) Insulin augmentation of 17β-hydroxylase activity is mediated by phosphatidyl inositol 3-kinase but not extracellular signal- regulated kinase-1/2 in human ovarian theca cells. Endocrinology 145:175–183
90. Nestler JE, Jakubowicz DJ, de Vargas AF et al (1998) Insulin stimulates testosterone biosynthesis by human thecal cells from women with polycystic ovary syndrome by activating its own receptor and using inositolglycan mediators as the signal transduction system. J Clin Endocrinol Metab 83:2001–2005
91. Barbieri RL, Makris A, Ryan KJ (1983) Effects of insulin on steroidogenesis in cultured porcine ovarian theca. Fertil Steril 40:237–241

92. Nestler JE, Strauss JF 3rd (1991) Insulin as an effector of human ovarian and adrenal steroid metabolism. Endocrinol Metab Clin North Am 20:807–823
93. Franks S, Gilling-Smith C, Watson H, Willis D (1999) Insulin action in the normal and polycystic ovary. Endocrinol Metab Clin North Am 28:361–378
94. Adashi EY, Hsueh AJ, Yen SS (1981) Insulin enhancement of luteinizing hormone and follicle-stimulating hormone release by cultured pituitary cells. Endocrinology 108:1441–1449
95. Micic D, Popovic V, Nesovic M et al (1988) Androgen levels during sequential insulin euglycemic clamp studies in patients with polycystic ovary disease. J Steroid Biochem 31:995–999
96. Dunaif A, Graf M (1989) Insulin administration alters gonadal steroid metabolism independent of changes in gonadotropin secretion in insulin-resistant women with the polycystic ovary syndrome. J Clin Invest 83:23–29
97. Nestler JE, Barlascini CO, Matt DW et al (1989) Suppression of serum insulin by diazoxide reduces serum testosterone levels in obese women with polycystic ovary syndrome. J Clin Endocrinol Metab 68:1027–1032
98. Plymate SR, Jones RE, Matej LA, Friedl KE (1988) Regulation of sex hormone binding globulin (SHBG) production in Hep G2 cells by insulin. Steroids 52:339–340
99. Nestler JE (1993) Sex hormone-binding globulin: a marker for hyperinsulinemia and/or insulin resistance? J Clin Endocrinol Metab 76:273–274
100. Dunaif A, Scott D, Finegood D et al (1996) The insulin-sensitizing agent troglitazone improves metabolic and reproductive abnormalities in the polycystic ovary syndrome. J Clin Endocrinol Metab 81:3299–3306
101. Azziz R, Ehrmann DA, Legro RS et al (2003) Troglitazone decreases adrenal androgen levels in women with polycystic ovary syndrome. Fertil Steril 79:932–937
102. Lawson MA, Jain S, Sun S et al (2008) Evidence for insulin suppression of baseline luteinizing hormone in women with polycystic ovarian syndrome and normal women. J Clin Endocrinol Metab 93:2089–2096
103. Eagleson CA, Bellows AB, Hu K et al (2003) Obese patients with polycystic ovary syndrome: evidence that metformin does not restore sensitivity of the gonadotropin-releasing hormone pulse generator to inhibition by ovarian steroids. J Clin Endocrinol Metab 88:5158–5162
104. Book C, Dunaif A (1999) Selective insulin resistance in the polycystic ovary syndrome. J Clin Endocrinol Metab 84(9):3110–3116
105. Diamanti-Kandarakis E, Dunaif A (2012) Insulin resistance and the polycystic ovary syndrome revisited: an update on mechanisms and implications. Endocr Rev 33(6):981–1030
106. Villa J, Pratley RE (2011) Adipose tissue dysfunction in polycystic ovary syndrome. Curr Diab Rep 11:179–184
107. Festa A, D'Agostino R Jr, Howard G et al (2000) Chronic subclinical inflammation as part of the insulin resistance syndrome: the Insulin Resistance Atherosclerosis Study (IRAS). Circulation 102:42–47
108. Kim HS, Ali O, Shim M et al (2007) Insulin-like growth factor binding protein-3 induces insulin resistance in adipocytes in vitro and in rats in vivo. Pediatr Res 61:159–164
109. Lee H, Oh J-Y, Sung Y-A (2013) Adipokines, insulin-like growth factor binding protein-3 levels, and insulin sensitivity in women with polycystic ovary syndrome. Korean J Intern Med 28:456–463

3.1 Endocrine Aspects of PCOS

Polycystic ovary syndrome (PCOS) is a chronic and self-perpetuating endocrine disorder, whose clinical, endocrine, and metabolic manifestations affect the whole life course of a patient. In PCOS, in fact, we can distinguish two sides of the same coin: endocrine and metabolic aspects.

A polycystic ovary appears enlarged with a thickened albuginea that has a porcelain appearance. In the subcapsular layer, there are many follicles measuring 2–10 mm in diameter, reduced number of granulosa cells, and a characteristic theca cell hyperplasia.

Thus, the fundamental abnormality is the presence of a raised number of follicles recruited with primary maturation block and increased atretic follicles.

3.1.1 Endocrine Pattern

3.1.1.1 Gonadotropins

PCOS is considered a normo-gonadotropic normo-estrogenic anovulatory disorder, but it is characterized by elevated LH serum concentrations with an inverted FSH/LH ratio [1].

PCOS follicles are present in large numbers, but they are arrested at an early to mid-developmental state and fail to mature even when they are exposed to normal FSH levels [2–4]. On the other hand, FSH levels do not increase during the early follicular phase to stimulate follicular maturation [5].

The resulting low estrogen and progesterone levels do not produce a negative feedback on LH secretion, and this is the major cause for the high serum LH concentrations in women with PCOS [6].

Despite these findings, gonadotropin levels have never been included in any of the diagnostic criteria for PCOS, especially because of the pulsatile nature of LH release [7–9].

© Springer International Publishing Switzerland 2015

M. Stracquadanio, L. Ciotta, *Metabolic Aspects of PCOS: Treatment with Insulin Sensitizers*, DOI 10.1007/978-3-319-16760-2_3

3.1.1.2 Sex Hormones

Hyperandrogenemia is the biochemical feature of PCOS. Elevated circulating androgen levels are observed in 80–90 % of women with oligomenorrhea [10].

In particular, a decreased SHBG (sex hormone-binding globulin) production with a consequent increase in free testosterone levels is reported. Furthermore, some authors suggest that, vice versa, SHBG levels are decreased in PCOS due to the effects of testosterone and insulin of decreasing hepatic production of SHBG [11, 12].

Ovaries are the main sources of increased androgens in PCOS, but even adrenal androgen excess is a common feature of the syndrome (approximately 20 % of PCOS women): an increased secretion of adrenocortical precursor steroids basally and in response to ACTH, such as pregnenolone, 17-hydroxyprogesterone (17-OHP), dehydroepiandrosterone (DHEA), and androstenedione (A), was demonstrated [13, 14].

It has been suggested that androgens enhance apoptosis in the granulosa cells of preantral and early antral follicles [15]. Moreover, a study found that the exposure to excessive androstenedione stimulates a premature luteinization of granulosa cells, most likely due to the loss of communication between the oocyte and the granulosa cell [16].

Due to the pulsatility of LH, only one blood parameter is not enough for the PCOS diagnosis, and there is no unanimous consensus on which androgen blood levels should be considered for a precise diagnosis (total or free testosterone, testosterone/SHBG ratio, or androstenedione). Usually, elevated levels of only DHEA or 17-OHP may exclude the diagnosis of PCOS [17].

3.1.1.3 Estrogens and Progesterone

Estradiol levels are constant, without the normal mid-cycle increase, while the levels of estrone are increased because of extraglandular aromatization of increased circulating androstenedione levels [18–20].

As a consequent of anovulation, progesterone levels are low in PCOS women; moreover, some authors reported that endometrial responsiveness to progesterone is reduced in PCOS women [21, 22] and that total endometrium PR (progesterone receptor) expression is higher in women with PCOS who have anovulation compared to women with PCOS who still ovulate [23].

Furthermore, the increased PR expression in epithelial cells is greater than that in stromal cells in women with PCOS, suggesting that lower binding of progesterone in stromal cells could lead to the promotion of estradiol-induced epithelial cell proliferation in PCOS women.

It has been hypothesized that lack of progesterone-induced and PR-mediated stromal cell proliferation could be a cause of progesterone resistance in PCOS patients [24].

3.1.1.4 AMH

Anti-Mullerian hormone (AMH) belongs to the transforming growth factor-β (TGF-β) superfamily. In women, AMH is produced by the granulosa cells of follicles from the stage of the primary follicle to the initial formation of the antrum. In female newborn, AMH is undetectable, but it increases gradually until puberty, remaining stable in the reproductive period [25].

Reduction of AMH levels in serum is the first indication of a decline in the follicular reserve of the ovaries. Moreover, AMH concentration remains stable during the cycle [26].

Since AMH level reflect the number of developing follicles, its measurement may be used as a marker of ovarian follicle damage in PCOS.

AMH levels are also probably related to the follicular arrest, during the selection process of the dominant follicle: AMH inhibits the recruitment of primordial follicles into the pool of growing follicles and decreases their receptiveness to FSH [27–29].

The first studies regarding AMH levels in PCOS women showed that AMH levels are higher than in healthy controls [30, 31]. Subsequent data indicated that these levels are related to increased number of small antral follicles of 2–5 mm diameter [32]: this correlation was found to be the strongest one [33].

The cause of the increased AMH production in PCOS is unknown: it is mainly ascribed to the increased production of AMH by each follicle, and it is not just a consequence of an increased follicle number, suggesting intrinsic granulosa cell dysregulation in PCOS [34, 35].

AMH levels are increased in proportion to PCOS clinical severity, as reflected by the antral follicle count [36, 37].

Furthermore, blood AMH appears to be associated with androgen levels, and so it has been proposed as a diagnostic marker for ovarian hyperandrogenism [38].

Some studies demonstrated, in fact, that AMH is positively correlated with total testosterone levels in normal-weight PCOS women [39].

AMH levels, as written before, decrease with age in women with normal ovulatory cycles; in PCOS women, this decline has a slower reduction rate, and it could be because of a decelerated ovarian aging, probably due to the negative effect of AMH on the recruitment of primordial follicles.

3.1.2   Clinical Endocrine Features

The clinical scenario of PCOS is very heterogeneous, and the symptoms are related to the ovarian dysfunction and hyperandrogenism.

This section describes the clinical characteristics of a PCOS woman, while the diagnostic pathway can be found in Chap. 6.

3.1.2.1 Menstrual Disorder

Since menarche, or after a short period, menstrual cycles show an irregular rhythm. In many cases they gradually distance themselves from each other, up to result in oligomenorrhea or in permanent amenorrhea. Menstrual dysfunction in women affected by PCOS may manifest in different ways, but the most common way is anovulation with erratic bleedings.

Although the presence of oligomenorrhea indicates ovulatory dysfunction, apparent eumenorrhea does not completely rule out anovulation [40].

Therefore, ovarian dysfunction usually manifests as oligomenorrhea/amenorrhea resulting from chronic oligo-ovulation/anovulation. The majority of women complaining oligomenorrhea (up to 80–90 %) are affected by PCOS [41].

A significant relationship between the degree of menstrual dysfunction and the degree of insulin resistance present was observed. After adjusting for BMI, age, and race, all PCOS subjects with menstrual cycles longer than 35 days had significantly higher mean HOMA-IR levels than controls, with those with cycle length longer than 3 months having the highest one [42]. Confirming these findings, it was reported also that among PCOS women insulin resistance was significantly worse in amenorrheic patients [43].

As consequent, prolonged anovulation can be the cause of dysfunctional uterine bleeding, which may mimic regular menstrual cycles.

In addition, the chronic anovulation implies prolonged estrogen excess (particularly in obese phenotype women) and lack of progesterone, resulting in atypical endometrial hyperplasia, which is the precursor of endometrial carcinoma [44, 45].

It is generally recommended that greater than four cycles per year may protect the endometrium [46].

3.1.2.2 Infertility

PCOS is the most common cause of anovulatory infertility: 90 % of women attending infertility clinic for anovulation disorder are affected by PCOS.

Despite these data, 60 % of women with PCOS are fertile, while time to conceive is often increased [41].

Moreover, infertile PCOS women are overweight in 90 % of cases.

Fifty percent of PCOS women experience recurrent pregnancy loss [47]: it is not clear whether these defects are caused by uterine dysfunction itself, by possible interrupted interaction between uterine cells and the developing embryo, or by insulin-related disorder.

The new guidelines suggest that PCOS is a risk factor for infertility only in the presence of oligo-ovulation or anovulation. However, there are no clear data about the fertility of PCOS patients who have normal ovulatory function [48].

3.1.2.3 Hirsutism

Hirsutism is defined as the presence of excessive terminal hairs in areas of the body that are androgen dependent and usually hairless or with limited hair growth, such as the face, chest, areolas, and abdomen [49].

Terminal hair is different from "vellus" hair, because the latter is the prolonged version of "lanugo" (the hair that covers fetuses and is shed gradually after birth) which covers all body surface except lips, palms, and soles; specifically, terminal hair is the pigmented, longer, coarser hair that covers the pubic and axillary areas, scalp, eyelashes, eyebrows, male body, and facial hair [50].

Hirsutism should be differentiated from hypertrichosis, which is the overgrowth of vellus in a nonsexual pattern distribution, usually related to persistence of the highly mitotic anagen phase of the hair cycle [51, 52].

Terminal hair growth requires androgen stimulation, specially testosterone and dihydrotestosterone (DHT) that can bind to the androgen receptor and promote hair follicle changes [50, 53].

Androgens, in fact, are the most significant hormones associated with hair growth modulation. They are necessary for terminal hair and sebaceous gland development and cause differentiation of pilosebaceous units into either a terminal hair follicle or a sebaceous gland. They are involved in keratinization, increased hair follicle size, hair fiber diameter, and the proportion of time that terminal hair spends in the anagen phase [54].

Thus, hyperandrogenemia is the cause of hirsutism, but the percentage of hair growth is not proportional to the degree of hyperandrogenism, supporting the important role for androgen receptor localization (keratinocytes, sebaceous glands, hair dermal papilla cells) and sensitivity in the development of hair patterns [55].

3.1.2.4 Acne and Seborrhea

Sebaceous glands are also androgen-dependent structures: sebocytes are highly sensitive to androgen signaling, which is worsened in PCOS, leading to the development of acne and seborrhea [56].

Androgens stimulate sebocyte proliferation (particularly in the mid-back, chin, and forehead) and secretion of sebum, which is a mixture of lipids including glycerides, squalene, free fatty acids (FFA), and cholesterol [57].

Local bacteria complicate the process by secreting lipolytic enzymes: they break down those triglycerides produced in the sebocyte; these FFAs are released into sebaceous ducts by apocrine glands, and they are responsible for the typical unpleasant odor [58].

3.1.2.5 Androgenic Alopecia

An opposite clinical feature is androgenic alopecia, which is a disorder characterized by miniaturized hair, due to an increased telogen/anagen ratio, and associated to genetic susceptibility related to increased 5α-reductase activity in the hair follicle. This increased enzymatic activity promotes the local conversion of testosterone into DHT, which has an increased androgen action.

Seventy percent of women with alopecia areata have PCOS with elevated levels of androstenedione and testosterone [59]. The balding pattern is mainly in the frontal and parietal scalp zones, while the occipital area has a great hair density [60].

3.1.2.6 Other Clinical Features

In rare cases, virilization patterns can be observed: they include increased size of clitoris, muscle mass hypertrophy, deep voice, temporal balding, and masculine aspect. In these cases, however, a lower ovarian or adrenal androgen-secreting neoplasm must be excluded.

Moreover, in PCOS women, nails could be affected by alterations, in the form of onycholysis [61] (separation of the nail plate from the nail bed caused by disruption of the onychocorneal band) and onychorrhexis [62] (splitting of nails in lengthway bridges). Nowadays the association of these nail diseases with hyperandrogenemia is not completely understood.

In literature, an unusual case of atypical oral hirsutism secondary to PCOS was described: a 19-year-old girl complained of the appearance of hairs on the sulcular epithelium of the retroincisor palatal papilla, relapsing after surgical excision. PCOS diagnosis was confirmed by clinical data (oligomenorrhea, face hirsutism, and acne), by serum studies, and by the symptom improvement after combined hormonal therapy [63].

3.1.2.7 PCOS and Thyroid Dysfunction

The most prevalent autoimmune disease in women is autoimmune thyroiditis (AIT), with a prevalence ranging from 4 to 21 %: it depends on age [64], diagnostic criteria, genetic differences, geographical origin, and iodine intake [65, 66]. In the past, a German study underlined the association between PCOS and AIT, but the pathogenesis of this relationship is not clear.

Few explanations were suggested, but none of these appears to be conclusive:

- Probable common genetic predisposition
- Imbalance between estrogens and progesterone, and the consequences of the stimulatory effect of estrogens on the immune system [67]
- Low-grade inflammatory state characteristic of PCOS

Recently, it has been shown that there is a higher prevalence of subclinical hypothyroidism in young women with PCOS compared with that reported for the general young women population [68].

Moreover, Mueller et al. [69] observed that PCOS patients with subclinical hypothyroidism had a higher prevalence of IR and a higher BMI.

3.2   Metabolic Aspects of PCOS

"Metabolic flexibility" is the capacity of the body to rapidly switch from predominant lipid oxidation (with high rates of fatty acid uptake in low-insulin conditions) to predominant glucose oxidation and storage with suppression of lipid oxidation in high-insulin conditions [70].

Few studies showed that obese and/or diabetic and/or insulin-resistant individuals, as compared with healthy lean individuals, have an impaired metabolic flexibility [71, 72].

Insulin resistance and the associated metabolic abnormalities are frequent findings in women with polycystic ovary syndrome [73].

Many women with PCOS meet the criteria for the metabolic syndrome (MS), as they report a higher incidence of hypertension, dyslipidemia, and visceral obesity [74].

Up to 43 % of nondiabetic PCOS women meet MS criteria before the end of their fourth decade, and most of them before the end of their third decade of life [75, 76].

This prevalence is four times higher than that observed in women aged 20–30 years and twice that of women between the ages of 30 and 40 years [77].

The prevalence of metabolic syndrome is similar across racial backgrounds [78].

Moreover, it was found that the prevalence of metabolic syndrome is higher in adolescent girls with PCOS: 37 % against 5 % of control non-PCOS girls [79].

The most common phenotypes in parents of adolescents with PCOS were found to be excessive weight and metabolic syndrome, particularly in fathers in whom the prevalence of MS and central obesity was 1.5–2-fold greater than expected in the general population [80].

The essential components of MS include insulin resistance or central obesity with at least two of hypertension, elevated triglycerides, decreased HDL-C levels, or elevated fasting glucose [81].

Insulin resistance, and consequent compensatory hyperinsulinemia, appears to be the central pathophysiologic mechanism that links PCOS to its metabolic disorders; in fact, few studies reported that PCOS women are more insulin resistant than controls who are matched for age and BMI [78].

Disturbance in the insulin's ability to bind to its receptor or in the transport mechanism across the cell membrane may lead to a state of a reduced sensitivity to insulin, or insulin resistance. Furthermore, pancreatic β-cell secretory dysfunction has also been reported [82, 83], and a reduction in hepatic insulin extraction contributes to the high insulin levels as well [84, 85].

Compensatory hyperinsulinemia is important in the development of metabolic abnormalities and also contributes to the high androgen levels, peculiar of PCOS women. As largely described in Chap. 2, it is important to remember that insulin binds to its receptor on the ovarian theca cell and it acts enhancing LH-stimulated androgen production [86]. Moreover, insulin can also act indirectly to raise free testosterone serum concentration by inhibiting the hepatic production of SHBG [12].

Although obesity is a major factor for the development of insulin resistance in PCOS, it is now well known that a component of insulin resistance is independent of body weight [87].

To underline the link between PCOS and metabolic syndrome, it is important to report that coronary heart disease, as well as cerebrovascular disease, is more common in postmenopausal PCOS patients. Persisting high androgen levels through the menopause, obesity, and maturity-onset diabetes mellitus are proposed as the main mechanisms accounting for the increased risk [88].

3.2.1 The Role of the Adipocyte in Linking PCOS to Metabolic Syndrome

Adipose tissue is nowadays considered not only a storage tissue but also a proper endocrine organ, metabolically active [89–92].

Adipose tissue responds to chronic changes in energy balance and nutrient content by altering the proliferation of pre-adipocytes, their differentiation into mature adipocytes, the growth and hypertrophy of adipocytes, and, finally, their apoptosis and necrosis [93]. In addition, rates of angiogenesis, extracellular matrix remodeling, and the relative distribution of the resident immune cell population in adipose tissue are modified in response to changes in nutritional status [94]. Thus, it is evident that adipose tissue acts as an enormous endocrine organ, secreting a variety of signaling molecules that regulate feeding behavior, energy spending, metabolism, reproduction, and endocrine and immune function [95].

Adipocytes secrete adiponectin, leptin, visfatin, tumor necrosis factor alpha (TNF-α), interleukin 6 (IL-6), plasminogen activator inhibitor-1 (PAI-1), resistin, and angiotensinogen: thus, adipose tissue results to be metabolically active [96, 97].

Adiponectin is a 244-amino acid protein that is expressed in white adipose tissue [98].

This adipokine expression within adipocytes is downregulated in obesity [99], and the result is that serum levels of adiponectin are inversely correlated with body weight [100].

Adiponectin has insulin-sensitizing, anti-atherogenic, and anti-inflammatory properties [101, 102]. It is well known that adiponectin has an important role in mediating the effects of increased fat mass on insulin sensitivity [103]: in fact, its low serum levels seem to be involved in conditions associated with insulin resistance, such as type II diabetes and obesity [104–106]; moreover, lower levels of serum adiponectin are present in PCOS women [107].

It also has been reported that adiponectin inhibits theca cell androgen production: suppressed levels of adiponectin may allow enhanced ovarian androgen production in PCOS women [108].

Leptin controls the fat disposition modulating its accumulation in the heart, liver, and kidneys; besides, it is involved in the control of vascular tone by producing a pressure action and opposing the NO-mediated relaxing function [109]: this could be associated with cardio-metabolic syndrome.

In humans, there is a strong association between the percentage of body fat and serum leptin levels [110]; some authors found that hyper-leptinemia has a positive relationship with insulin-resistant PCOS women [111], even if more studies are needed to confirm it.

Hyper-leptinemia seems to lower the sensitivity of dominant ovarian follicles to insulin-like growth factor 1 (IGF-1), which is implicated in the mechanism of anovulation [112].

Visfatin is a multifunctional protein that plays a number of roles including the regulation of metabolism and inflammation, and it is also involved in the insulin resistance mechanism [113, 114].

Few recent studies have demonstrated that visfatin levels are significantly higher in PCOS women comparing to the healthy controls [115], even when considering only the overweight and obese subgroups [116].

It has been demonstrated that in women with PCOS, adipocyte diameter is 25 % greater than the diameter of adipocytes taken from obese control women with comparable BMI: adipocyte seems to be hypertrophic [117].

Adipocyte hypertrophy in PCOS may be a consequence of variations in storage and/or adipocyte lipolytic capacity. Thus, obesity in women with PCOS is mainly characterized by an increase in fat cell size (hypertrophic obesity) rather than an increase in fat cell number (hyperplastic obesity) [118].

In PCOS subcutaneous adipocytes, there is a reduced catecholamine-mediated lipolysis [119], and maybe there is an implication of testosterone as a possible contributory factor in this process [120]. Greater lipolysis within visceral adipocytes results in hepatic insulin resistance through increased hepatic influx of portal free fatty acids; reduced lipolysis within subcutaneous adipocytes is likely to be one explanation for adipocyte hypertrophy and consequent insulin resistance [108].

Studies on the molecular insulin signaling pathways within PCOS adipocytes have demonstrated that the number of insulin receptors and the affinity of these receptors for insulin are normal [121–123]. Moreover, there are evidences that, in PCOS adipocytes, basal auto-phosphorylation of the insulin receptor β-subunit is normal, but insulin-dependent auto-phosphorylation is significantly reduced [123].

The existing literature suggests a large number of possible defective post-insulin receptor molecular mechanisms that may explain adipocyte's insulin resistance in PCOS, although the actual mechanism involved and the determinants of adipocyte size in PCOS are not fully understood [108].

In the past, Danforth hypothesized that the inability to differentiate sufficient new subcutaneous adipocytes in response to chronic excessive energy intake may explain the metabolic dysfunction observed in some obese women: thus, a deficiency in either the proliferation or differentiation capacity of adipocytes leads to the redistribution of fat from subcutaneous to visceral depots and also to other tissues such as the liver and skeletal muscle, where the ectopic fat causes insulin resistance [124].

Furthermore, steroidogenic activity within the adipocyte plays a crucial role in the development of PCOS, particularly the hyperandrogenemia associated with PCOS: this could be the link between obesity and hyperandrogenemic features [108].

Although the predominant source of raised androgens in PCOS women is ovarian, adrenal androgen secretion is also important [125]; moreover, peripheral conversion of androstenedione and DHEAS accounts for up to 50 % of circulating testosterone in PCOS women, and the major peripheral site is the adipose tissue [126].

The 5α-reductase enzyme is present in the adipocyte cell and it converts testosterone into the more potent 5α-dihydrotestosterone (DHT), and it is also involved in the catabolism of cortisol [125].

It is supposed that PCOS women have enhanced peripheral 5α-reductase activity compared with age and BMI-matched control women [127–130]. This causes an increased production of DHT, increased catabolism of cortisol, and consequent reduced feedback of cortisol on the pituitary corticotroph cells [125].

Furthermore, increasing adipose tissue mass is directly associated with increasing levels of angiotensin II from the increased secretion of angiotensinogen by adipose tissue; this increase could contribute to hypertension and worsen insulin resistance [131].

On the other hand, few molecules secreted by adipocytes are involved in macrophage function, including monocyte chemoattractant protein-1 (MCP-1), macrophage migration inhibitory factor, and macrophage inflammatory protein (MIP)-1α which are upregulated in obesity [132]. Adipose tissue resident macrophages from obese women are activated and also express few proteins such as MIP-1α, MCP-1, and related inflammatory cytokines, which may play a role in the development of obesity-induced insulin resistance [118]. Most adipose tissue TNF-α, inducible nitric oxide synthase, and IL-6 seem to be expressed by adipose tissue macrophages, rather than adipocyte [94]. IL-6 inhibits lipoprotein lipase activity, stimulates aromatase activity, and increases the hepatic production of triglycerides [133]. IL-6 is stimulated by TNF-α: the latter stimulates C-reactive protein (CRP), which is highly associated with obesity, insulin resistance, and endothelial dysfunction; PCOS women seem to have higher levels of CRP [134, 135] and, specifically, of hs-CRP (high-sensitive CRP), which is the most specific marker [136].

Elevation of these inflammatory markers is in accord with the hypothesis that atheroma formation is primarily an inflammatory condition [137].

3.2.2   The Role of Vitamin D in the Development of Metabolic Syndrome in PCOS Women

Few evidences suggest that vitamin D deficiency could be a causal factor in the pathogenesis of metabolic syndrome in PCOS women [138].

It is well known that the vitamin D receptor gene regulates 3 % of the human genome, including genes essential for glucose and lipid metabolism and blood pressure regulation [139–141].

In fact, clinical studies had reported insulin resistance and obesity association with hypovitaminosis D [138, 142, 143].

The mechanism underlying the association between low vitamin D levels and insulin resistance is not completely assumed. The suggested hypotheses are the following:

- Vitamin D may have a positive effect on insulin action by stimulating the expression of insulin receptor and improving insulin receptiveness for glucose transport [140].
- Vitamin D regulates extracellular and intracellular calcium, which is important for insulin-mediated intracellular processes in insulin-responsive tissue (skeletal muscle and adipose tissue) [140].
- Vitamin D has a modulating effect on the immune system, so hypovitaminosis D might have a pro-inflammatory action, which is associated with insulin resistance [144, 145].

Moreover, it is not fully understood whether vitamin D insufficiency results from obesity and/or whether obesity is a consequence of hypovitaminosis D.

Despite there is not a clear consensus regarding its optimal value, a level of 30 ng/ml indicates a sufficient vitamin D status [139]; concentrations of 20–30 ng/ml are considered as vitamin D insufficiency, while a level less than 20 ng/ml represents a vitamin D deficiency [139].

In a recent study, 72.8 % of PCOS women showed values below the abovementioned normal cutoff; a significant association of hypovitaminosis with increased levels of both fasting and stimulated glucose and insulin, elevated HOMA-IR, and incidence of MS was demonstrated [146].

Furthermore, vitamin D levels were significantly lower in hirsute woman, as shown in previous study [138, 147]. For example, distress caused by the excessive hair might lead to hypovitaminosis D because of the decreased sun exposure of hirsute women.

Vitamin D receptor is present in keratinocytes of the outer root sheath as well as in cells of the bulge, indicating an important role of vitamin D in hair follicle cycling [144].

3.2.3   Metabolic Syndrome and Associated Disorders

3.2.3.1 Visceral Obesity

The prevalence of obesity in PCOS varies from approximately 10 % up to 50 % [148, 149].

A likely explanation for the mechanism underlying the development of obesity in women with PCOS is the combined effect of a genetic predisposition to obesity in the context of an "obesogenic" environment (poor diet and reduced exercise). The development of obesity in PCOS patients, in turn, amplifies and unmasks the biochemical and clinical abnormalities characteristic of this condition [125].

Obese PCOS women have lower levels of SHBG, DHEAS, DHEA, IGF-1, and HDL and higher LDL compared with the nonobese PCOS controls [150].

It is important to underline that all overweight/obese people are not insulin resistant, and those who are insulin resistant are not all obese.

Previous researches have studied the importance of fat distribution patterns as risk factor for cardiovascular and metabolic disease such as diabetes mellitus [151, 152].

In fact, gluteo-femoral obesity is less associated with insulin resistance than is central or android obesity [153].

The gynoid type of fat distribution, where fat accumulates around the hips, thighs, and buttocks, is developed during female puberty and is maintained during the fertile phase [152, 154].

Approximately 50–60 % of PCOS women are characterized by a so-called "android" distribution of body fat, whereby a disproportionate quantity of adipose tissue is distributed in the visceral depot [155, 156]: they have a higher trunk/periphery fat ratio [157].

This upper body fat distribution has been explained mainly by androgen excess [158], and it is an independent factor of BMI [159]: the pathogenic mechanisms involved have not yet been defined.

In women affected by PCOS, android body fat distribution per se contributes to hyperandrogenemia, through its adverse effects on insulin sensitivity and consequent ovarian co-gonadotropic effects of hyperinsulinemia.

Hyperinsulinemia itself contributes to obesity by the anabolic effect on fat metabolism through the adipogenesis process: the result is an increased uptake of glucose into adipocytes, the production of triglycerides, and the inhibition of hormone-sensitive lipase [160].

Therefore, there is a vicious cycle in which android fat produces android fat and exacerbates the predisposition toward weight gain [125].

Visceral fat, or abdominal fat, is metabolically distinct from subcutaneous fat; it is resistant to the anti-lipolytic effects of insulin and releases excessive amounts of free fatty acids, which leads to IR in the liver and muscle. In response to it, in the liver, there is an increased gluconeogenesis, and in the muscle there is an inhibition of insulin-mediated glucose uptake [161–163].

Excess fat itself contributes to IR at the level of the adipocyte: when fat cells become too large, they are unable to store additional lipids, and then, fat is stored in the muscle, liver, and beta cells of the pancreas [164]. Visceral fat also produces excess of 11-beta-hydroxysteroid-dehydrogenase-1 [163], an enzyme that converts inactive cortisone to the biochemically active cortisol: the latter is able to promote central adiposity and IR [165].

3.2.3.2 Dyslipidemia

The probability of a metabolic disorder in families of PCOS patients is 2.7-fold higher compared with normal families, and the relative risk for developing dyslipidemia is 1.8 [166].

Dyslipidemia is reported in up to 70 % of patients who have PCOS, according to the National Cholesterol Education Program (NCEP) guidelines [167].

Dyslipidemia in PCOS women seems to be well understood, but which are the determinant factors of this pattern? Insulin, estrogens, and androgens are each well known to alter lipoprotein lipid metabolism [168]. All of them influence hepatic lipase activity, which is important in reductive metabolism of intermediate-density lipoproteins to small dense LDL particles; greater activity of this enzyme was found in PCOS women [169].

Insulin stimulates lipogenesis in arterial and adipose tissues via an increased production of acetyl CoA and the entry of glucose and triglycerides [170].

PCOS women have higher Apo-CIII levels compared to non-PCOS controls [171]: understanding its metabolism is helpful to deeply comprehend the pathophysiology of dyslipidemia in PCOS.

In states of IR, it has been shown an increased synthesis of ApoC-III [172]: in PCOS, with central obesity more free fatty acids flow into the portal vein and more glucose is available, causing altered apolipoprotein lipid metabolism. The ratio of ApoC-II/CII is increased and triglycerides carried in VLDL are broken into more atherogenic small LDL particles, which circulate and enter the arterial wall to initiate inflammation. With elevated triglycerides, VLDL lipolysis is slowed, causing greater residence time for ApoB, remnant particles, LD particles and small LDL-particles. ApoC-I, recently shown to be elevated in normal-weight PCOS women, blocks lipoprotein lipase, cholesterol ester transferase, lecithin cholesterol acyltransferase, VLDL receptors and LDL receptors in the liver. All of these events lead to more exposure of the blood vessel wall to entry of atherogenic particles with the potential for setting inflammation and atherogenesis. [168]

Moreover, insulin increases the levels of HMG-CoA reductase, the rate-limiting enzyme in the synthesis of cholesterol: this effect may contribute to the raised cholesterol level, which is also a feature of hyperinsulinemia [173].

Hyperandrogenism and lipid metabolism are closely related: in fact, it has been observed that testosterone has a deleterious effect on lipid profile [174, 175]. Testosterone has been involved in lowering HDL-C levels, an effect attributed to the upregulation of two genes implicated in the catabolism of HDL: scavenger receptor B1 (SR-B1) and hepatic lipase [176].

The most common lipid profile found in PCOS individuals is characterized by [176–182]:

- Increased levels of LDL cholesterol (especially raised amounts of types III and IV small LDL particles [176])
- Increased VLDL cholesterol
- Increased triglycerides
- Reduced levels of HDL cholesterol (particularly decreased HDL2, the most anti-atherogenic HDL subtype)

Particularly, a study has demonstrated that the incidence of high triglycerides increased progressively from the lean to the obese PCOS women, and the incidence of low HDL was three times higher in the overweight than in the lean PCOS subgroup [183].

HDL-C has several functions: inhibition of LDL-C oxidation, transport of cholesterol from peripheral cells to the liver, anti-apoptotic effects, and antithrombotic and antioxidant effects. For this reason, low HDL-C is considered an independent cardiovascular risk factor: thus, women with PCOS may have a higher cardiovascular risk than normal women at the same BMI level [184].

Furthermore, these lipid disorders are exacerbated among those women who develop glucose intolerance in association with PCOS; in fact, 88 % of women with PCOS and IGT or type II diabetes have an abnormal lipid profile, compared with 58 % of women with PCOS and normal glucose tolerance [177].

Even PCOS adolescents have less favorable blood lipid profiles, with higher LDL-C and lower levels of HDL-C, and they appear to be more insulin resistant than their peer control with higher fasting C peptide levels [185].

3.2.3.3 NAFLD (Nonalcoholic Fatty Liver Disease)

NAFLD represents a disease spectrum ranging from steatosis hepatitis (SH or NAFL) to nonalcoholic steato-hepatitis (NASH), characterized by hepatocyte injury, inflammation, and fibrosis, which can progress to cirrhosis in 25 % of cases, with its long-term complications, such as portal hypertension, liver failure, and hepatocellular carcinoma [186].

The hepatic steatosis is histopathologically characterized by the accumulation of triglycerides, both in the form of macro- and microvesicles, in more than 5 % of hepatocytes. These "fatty hepatocytes" are usually peri-venular located, and they are mainly present at the level of the "portal areas." The pool of fatty acids available for the synthesis of triglycerides is related to the balance between their formation and utilization. The deposition of triglycerides into the hepatocytes depends on both of these reactions: thus, the development of a fatty liver is the consequence of a dysfunction in different metabolic pathways.

There are important relationships between peripheral insulin resistance and hepatic fat deposition. High intake of calories in sedentary individuals who are genetically susceptible induces a state of IR, which involves an increased lipolysis, as a result of free fatty acid and TNF-α circulating levels and of lower levels of adiponectin: this increases both insulin resistance and circulating levels of free fatty acids. The raised fat deposition in the liver induces insulin resistance by itself, activating abnormal insulin intracellular signals. Both these processes lead to an increased hepatic insulin resistance and deposition of fatty acids.

These events, in turn, cause a dysregulation of some sterol regulatory proteins (SREBP-1C) and, probably, of ghrelin. This pathogenic mechanism is responsible for inducing a de novo lipogenesis in the liver.

Thus, it is well evident that NAFLD is a complex and multifactorial disease, and it is currently the most common cause of liver disease and high enzyme levels in clinical practice. Probably a state of IR plays critical part in both the development and progression of the liver disease. It seems that an important role is assumed by oxidative stress and some adipokines, such as TNF-α and adiponectin. Moreover, the nature of the epidemic NAFLD, as well as its clear association with obesity and metabolic syndrome, makes the altered lifestyle and a sedentary lifestyle conditioning factors in the development of this disease even in teenagers [187].

Even if liver biopsy is the "gold standard" for distinguishing between simple steatosis and NASH, and for disease severity assessment, the diagnosis of fatty liver is clinically performed by ultrasound:

1. Absent: the echogenicity of the liver parenchyma is greater than or equal to that of the cortex of the kidney; there is a clear view of the intrahepatic venous system.
2. Mild fatty liver: slight increase of fine echoes in the liver parenchyma with normal visualization of the intrahepatic venous circulation.
3. Moderate hepatic steatosis: moderate and widespread increase of fine echoes in the liver parenchyma with impaired visualization of intrahepatic venous system.
4. Severe fatty liver: marked increased echogenicity of the liver parenchyma with deficiency or absence of visualization of intrahepatic venous circulation [187].

The extent of steatosis is related to the degree of insulin resistance [188].

Elevated liver enzymes have been used as a noninvasive surrogate marker of NAFLD, provided that other potential causes of liver disease (chronic viral hepatitis, alcohol-induced liver disease, etc.) have been excluded.

The typical pattern of abnormal liver biochemical profile includes increased serum aminotransferases, with a predominant increase of alanine aminotransferase (ALT), relative to aspartate aminotransferase (AST), accompanied by elevated γ-glutamyl transpeptidase levels (γ-GT) [189, 190].

Elevated ALT, above the level of 35 U/l, has been detected in 30 % of overweight/obese PCOS women [191, 192].

Both adult and pediatric patients with NASH are commonly asymptomatic. Rarely, patients may present with persistent right upper quadrant pain or chronic pain in the umbilical region. On physical examination, more than 90 % of patients with NASH are found to be obese, and acanthosis nigricans has been reported in 36–49 % of patients [193].

A number of studies have demonstrated a high risk of hepatic steatosis in women with PCOS [187, 192, 194–196].

A recent study has shown that women with hyperandrogenic PCOS have evidence of increased liver fat, compared with PCOS women with normal androgens or with healthy controls [197].

In one of our studies, an elevated percentage of NAFLD both in lean and obese women, with a low rate of hepatomegaly (8.3 %) and 15 % of elevated liver enzymes, was found. In fact, liver enzyme impairment is not always associated to the presence of NAFLD, and vice versa [187].

Moreover, in contrast to what happens in other population subgroup where only a minority of patients who suffer from NAFLD progress to NASH, the prevalence of advanced liver disease (NASH with fibrosis) in women with PCOS is higher [192, 198] even in the adolescent population [199].

For these reasons, from a clinical point of view, it seems advisable to closely follow women with PCOS and insulin resistance, particularly in the presence of body weight alterations.

3.2.3.4 Hypertension

Hyperinsulinemia may contribute to the hypertension (which is part of the metabolic syndrome) by several mechanisms:

- Stimulating the renin–angiotensin–aldosterone system and consequently increasing renal sodium reabsorption [200, 201]
- Causing an increased intracellular sodium and calcium [202]
- Inducing vasoconstriction by stimulation of the sympathetic nervous system [203–205]
- Stimulating the release of IGF-1 that may contribute to the development of hypertension by causing vascular smooth muscle hypertrophy [137]

The prevalence of hypertension in PCOS women increases with BMI as independent factor [206].

Women with PCOS were found to have an increased left atrial size and left ventricular mass index, with a reduced left ventricular ejection fraction [207], which is directly related to the degree of insulin resistance; this finding may represent early remodeling as a prelude to overt cardiac dysfunction [208].

The results of many studies are controversial: in a few of them, both systolic and diastolic blood pressures are normal [124, 209–212], while in other studies, mean arterial pressures and ambulatory systolic pressures are elevated in women with PCOS compared with non-PCOS controls [212].

PCOS patients appear to be at increased risk for developing hypertension, at least later in life if it doesn't occur during the reproductive age.

For menopausal or climacteric women with a previous history of PCOS, this prevalence varies from 28.1 to 39 % [209, 213], while for patients who are in their third or fourth decades of life, the prevalence varies from 3.8 to 22 % [213–215].

This difference of prevalence according to the age range is probably a consequence of aging itself.

3.2.3.5 Diabetes

PCOS women are at high risk of progression to impaired glucose metabolism and type II diabetes; a family history of type II diabetes is present in a large percentage of women affected by PCOS, suggesting the important role of the genetic pattern in the development of the syndrome.

Generally, glucose levels remain normal in PCOS despite insulin resistance, because of compensatory pancreatic β-cell insulin production resulting in hyperinsulinemia. However, some patients have a genetic susceptibility to pancreatic β-cell failure and, over time, develop elevations in glucose when pancreatic β-cell insulin production can no longer overcome the insulin resistance [216].

A study reported that 35 % of patients with PCOS had impaired glucose tolerance (IGT) and 10 % had type II diabetes (T2DM) by the age of 40 [217].

A very recent study showed that the conversion rate from IGT to T2DM in women with PCOS was higher than that in the general population of women with IGT: 2–10.75 % vs 1–7 % per year [218].

Moreover, it was clearly shown that the risk for IGT or T2DM in women with PCOS was amplified (fourfold increase) in the presence of obesity, highlighting the role of patient weight in the development of glucose metabolism disorders [218].

A Korean study found that nonobese patients with PCOS presented a higher prevalence of elevated glycated hemoglobin than nonobese controls [219].

Both IGT and T2DM are very significant cardiovascular risk factors in women. Once the diagnosis of diabetes is made, the relative risk of cardiovascular disease in women increases fourfold to sevenfold, with a greater risk of cardiovascular disease and heart failure compared to men with diabetes [220].

With regard to mortality rates, diabetes may be a more prominent contributing cause of death in women with PCOS compared with the general population [221].

3.2.3.6 Obstructive Sleep Apnea

Obstructive sleep apnea (OSA) is a known cardiovascular risk factor and is one of the major causes of chronic sleep disruption. It is characterized by episodic partial or complete upper airway obstruction during sleep, leading to intermittent hypoxia, sleep fragmentation, and a reduction in the quantity of deep non-rapid eye movement (NREM) sleep or "slow wave sleep" (SWS). This alteration has been associated with cortisol levels rising [222].

OSA has been independently related to glucose intolerance and insulin resistance even after adjustments for obesity and age [223–227], and PCOS women are 5–30 times more likely to have this disorder compared to controls [167, 176, 228–231].

The mechanism by which PCOS increases the risk of OSA remains unclear.

The high prevalence of this disorder cannot be fully attributed to excess adiposity, as reported in some studies: in two studies the severity of OSA did not correlate with BMI [229–231], and in another one, even after controlling for BMI, women with PCOS were 30 times more likely to have breathing disorders during sleep and 9 times more likely to have daytime sleepiness than the control women [230].

On the other hand, according to a recent study, nonobese women with PCOS do not seem to be at increased risk of OSA: this raised risk is only present among the obese women [232]. Other studies have also indicated that obese women with PCOS who have OSA are more insulin resistant compared to obese women with PCOS who do not have OSA [231, 233, 234].

Insulin resistance, in fact, seems to be a stronger predictor of OSA, more than age, BMI, or circulating testosterone concentration [229]: the role of androgen elevation in the pathogenesis of OSA in women with PCOS remains controversial [229, 230].

Another potential pathogenic mechanism is the "low progesterone theory": it has been estimated that the upper airway resistance is lower during the luteal phase, when usually progesterone is higher, compared with follicular phase when progesterone is low [235]. Progesterone promotes its effects through direct stimulation of respiratory drive [236] and enhancement of the upper airway dilator muscle activity [237] by which it reduces airway resistance. Because women with PCOS have usually anovulatory cycles, and so circulating progesterone concentrations reflect the constantly lower levels of the follicular phase, this may contribute to the high prevalence of OSA in PCOS [238].

3.2.3.7 Plasma Viscosity and Pro-thrombotic State

In healthy individuals, there is equilibrium between the hemostatic coagulation and fibrinolytic systems: thrombosis results from an imbalance between these complex systems [239]. The hemostatic system plays an important role in cardiovascular disease: for example, acute events often precipitate by thrombosis developing on a ruptured arterial plaque.

Plasma viscosity is an important hemorheologic variable, and it is mainly determined by several macromolecules, such as fibrinogen, immunoglobulins, and lipoproteins [240].

Plasma viscosity is an indicator of blood flow in the network of small blood vessels that constitute microcirculation. An elevated plasma viscosity indicates increased resistance to blood flow in most tissues of the body [241].

Chronic hyperviscosity is able to impair microcirculation and promote target organ damage [242], and it is considered an independent predictor of cardiac events and mortality [243–245].

In a recent study, plasma viscosity is not connected to serum androgen levels, but it is correlated with serum fasting insulin and cholesterol levels, which appear to be higher in hirsute women compared to the matched for age and BMI healthy controls [246, 247].

Mild or chronic hyperviscosity is very frequent in older patients with metabolic syndrome (MS) and insulin resistance (IR) [248–250]. A deterioration of plasma viscosity was found to be present even in young, slightly overweight, PCOS women with IR who might be exposed to the same risk factors for cardiovascular diseases as older obese patients with MS. For this reason, plasma viscosity might be useful in the assessment of cardiovascular risk in young women with PCOS, in addition to plasma cholesterol and atherogenic index (triglycerides/HDL-C) [247].

Hyperinsulinemia contributes to the pro-thrombotic state by reducing fibrinolysis and raising the level of PAI-1 (plasminogen activator inhibitor-1). The increase of the latter in PCOS women seems to be independent of BMI: elevated levels, in fact, were observed in lean PCOS women too [137].

The procoagulant state is, in part, due to platelet hyperactivity, which was observed in lean women with PCOS [251] and in type II diabetic patients [252]. Why?

Platelets are involved in acute thrombosis, initiation of atheroma, and modulation of inflammatory responses, and they contribute to endothelial dysfunction [253]. Platelets are able to adhere to intact activated endothelium in the absence of exposed extracellular matrix proteins [254]. These adherent platelets could have a critical role in atherogenesis phenomenon, by secreting chemokines CCL5, CXCL4, and IL-1 [255].

Normally, platelet activation is counterbalanced by inhibitory signaling cascades that are activated by endothelial-derived NO and prostacyclin (PGI2), which modulate excessive activation [256].

Platelet hyperactivity seems to be related to acute hypertriglyceridemia: in fact, high levels of triglycerides might decrease the production of endothelial NO and PGI2, acting as a stimulator of platelet activation [257].

3.2.3.8 Chronic Inflammation, Endothelial Function, and Atherosclerosis

The presence of cardiovascular risk factors such as obesity, insulin resistance, and dyslipidemia may predispose PCOS women to coronary heart disease, but the topic is still controversial [137].

One of the early signs of cardiovascular lesions is the endothelial injury [258]. Several authors have reported precocious anatomical and functional arterial changes in PCOS women [259–261].

A positive correlation was demonstrated between abnormal endothelial function and testosterone levels in hyperandrogenic insulin-resistant women [262], while others have reported no differences for increased cardiovascular risk [263].

Mechanisms involved in the development of endothelial dysfunction could be the following:

- Reduced synthesis and release of nitric oxide (NO) [264].
- Enhanced inactivation of NO after its release from endothelial cells [265].
- Enhanced synthesis of vasoconstricting agents [266].
- Insulin itself acts directly on the vascular endothelium and the smooth muscle cells by a hypertrophic effect.

Insulin stimulates both endothelin-1 and NO activity in the skeletal muscle circulation: an imbalance between the release of these factors may be involved in the pathophysiology of endothelial dysfunction.

In normal women, aging per se is associated with progressive attenuation of nitric oxide signaling; in PCOS women, these changes are present in early adult life, predisposing polycystic ovarian syndrome patients to premature atherosclerosis; in fact, high levels of plasma ADMA were found: endogenous NO synthase inhibitor N^G-N^G-dimethyl-L-arginine (ADMA) is a biochemical marker/mediator of endothelial dysfunction [267].

Furthermore, the important role of obesity in the mechanism of endothelial dysfunction in PCOS women was shown: in humans, adiponectin enhances endothelium-dependent and endothelium-independent vasodilatation, reduces levels of TNF-α, and diminishes its effects on endothelial cells [268, 269]. This, in turn, reduces neointimal thickening and proliferation of smooth muscle cells, inhibits endothelial cell proliferation and migration, inhibits endothelial effects of oxidized LDL, and attenuates growth factor effects on smooth muscle cells [270–273].

Nowadays, it is clear that PCOS is a pro-inflammatory state, and emerging data suggest that chronic low-grade inflammation supports the development of metabolic aberration and ovarian dysfunction [274, 275].

CRP is the most reliable circulating marker of chronic low-grade inflammation in PCOS [276]. Recently, CRP was found to be a direct promoter of the atherosclerotic processes and endothelial cell inflammation leading to atherothrombosis [137].

CRP has a direct role in the vascular inflammatory process stimulating the release of inflammatory cytokines and increasing endothelial expression of cellular adhesion molecules, which mediate leukocyte migration [277].

Findings of a study suggest that increased cardiovascular risk may be seen in 83.3 % of the PCO women with CRP >2.42 mg/l [278].

CRP values <1 mg/l are considered low risk, 1–3 mg/l are considered intermediate risk, and 3–10 mg/l are considered high risk for cardiovascular disease [279].

Anatomic evidence of early coronary and other vascular diseases in PCOS women has been reported: it seems that PCOS patients have increased carotid artery intima-media thickness (IMT) compared with age-matched control women [280].

Increased IMT has been linked to cardiovascular risk factors including dyslipidemia and obesity, and it is considered an independent predictor of stroke and myocardial infarction [78].

The role of hs-CRP in predicting increased carotid intima-media thickness is not independent of BMI in PCOS [280].

Coronary artery calcification, another marker of atherosclerosis, is more common in women with PCOS than in controls, even after adjustment for the effects of age and BMI [281–283].

3.2.4 Role of Insulin Resistance in Infertility and Pregnancy Outcome

As pointed out previously, PCOS is the most common cause of anovulatory infertility: 90 % of women attending infertility clinic for anovulation disorder are affected by PCOS, and the rising incidence of PCOS women who have been subjected to IVF had permitted several studies on their oocyte quality.

On the other hand, without considering IVF pregnancies, increased incidence of pregnancy complications such as miscarriage, gestational diabetes mellitus (GDM), preeclampsia, preterm delivery, and perinatal mortality has been reported in polycystic ovary syndrome (PCOS) pregnancies: an increase of two to four times was noticed [284].

3.2.4.1 Oocyte Quality

Obesity has been associated with lower levels of anti-Mullerian hormone (AMH), which can indicate a decrease in ovarian reserve or available secondary follicles in obese women [285]. Obese women also have lower levels of LH than normal-weight women, and an independent positive association between LH and AMH levels has been demonstrated [36]. Moreover, women with BMI >25 have lower excretion of gonadotropins and luteal phase progesterone metabolites, implying that obesity has a negative effect on corpus luteum function [286].

Studies directly examining oocyte quality have suggested that an altered maternal metabolic environment results in an abnormal follicular fluid microenvironment, with a subsequent poor oocyte and embryo quality.

Women with higher BMI had increased levels of insulin, lactate, triglycerides, and CRP in the follicular fluid and decreased levels of SHBG [287], indicating that the maternal metabolic environment has a direct effect on the ovarian follicular microenvironment [288].

The increased CRP in the follicular fluid indicates inflammation and increased oxidative stress, with consequent decreased developmental potential in the oocyte [287, 289]. A recent analysis has showed that obese PCOS women have smaller oocyte size compared with the control group [290], but nowadays the effect of oocyte size on developmental competence and pregnancy outcome is unknown.

3.2.4.2 Recurrent Pregnancy Loss

Recurrent pregnancy loss (RPL) is defined by two or more failed pregnancies and it is found in 1–5 % of couples during pregnancy, and 50 % of these cases remain unexplained [291]. The incidence rate between PCOS and recurrent miscarriage is not clear because of its large variation in different studies [292–295]. Some authors have reported that PCOS women have a 33 % chance of spontaneous abortion [293, 296].

The following are the two most reasonable mechanisms:

1. LH hypersecretion: inappropriate LH secretion during the follicular stage might cause premature oocyte maturation through inhibition of oocyte maturation inhibitor [297]. The hyperandrogenemia secondary to increased LH levels impacts on ovarian folliculogenesis, resulting in abnormal granulosa cell function and follicular atresia.

   Moreover, the abnormal endocrine environment might exert an influence on the endometrium, and the ultimate cause of miscarriage could be secondary to endometrial non-receptivity [298].

   It has also been suggested that PCOS is associated with an endometrial inflammatory reaction affecting implantation on the basis of raised levels of CRP [280, 299, 300]. In fact, the low-grade chronic inflammation status could be the expression of an abnormal immune regulation during pregnancy, with an increase in the frequency and the extent of immune-mediated placental pathologies that probably reduce the maternal immunological permissiveness to trophoblastic invasion and placentation in PCOS women [301, 302].

A recent study demonstrated an increased incidence of placental lesions such as chronic villitis and intervillositis [302].

2. Hyperinsulinemia has been proposed as the route for the effect of obesity on some reproductive abnormalities, probably through its effect on androgen production. Hyperinsulinemia seems to adversely affect the preimplantation environment by decreasing the expression of glycodelin and IGF-binding protein-1 [303], which may play a role in inhibiting the endometrial immune response of the embryo and facilitating adhesion processes at the feto-maternal interface [291].

   In a few studies, a positive relationship between HOMA2-IR and spontaneous abortion suggests IR as a significant predictor of pregnancy loss [304, 305].

   Recent studies consider the occurrence of hypofibrinolysis associated with high plasminogen activator inhibitor-1 (PAI-1) the reason for RPL [306, 307]. The effects of elevated PAI-1 may also be worsen by elevated homocysteine [308]; in fact, some studies propose a possible association between insulin resistance (IR) and hyperhomocysteinemia (HHcy) [309] due to a documented increased incidence of the latter in PCOS women [310]. Apart from the thrombogenic effect of elevated Hcy on pregnant PCOS women (resulting in microthrombus formation causing placental dysfunction), recent findings have implicated the adverse effect of HHcy on the defect in folliculogenesis [311], embryo quality [312], oocyte number, and maturation [313].

   A recent study clearly showed that PCOS and pregnancy affect the hemostatic indices independently; the significant interaction between PCOS and pregnancy only affects the activity levels of factor (F)VIII and factor (F)X. As already highlighted, when nonpregnant women with PCOS become pregnant, they are likely to be in a more pro-thrombotic state than healthy women who get pregnant, as the activities of FVIII and FX and the levels of Von Willebrand factor (WF) and PAI-1 (which are involved in the coagulation cascade) are significantly higher in PCOS pregnant women [284].

   Moreover, as well explained previously, there is a strict connection between hyperinsulinemia and adipose tissue function in PCOS women. The already cited adiponectin and adiponectin receptors are involved in the female reproductive tract; the mechanism by which adiponectin system regulates implantation and early pregnancy remains unknown. It has been reported that a failure on adiponectin system leads to a suboptimal uterine decidualization and pregnancy loss in obesity and PCOS [314].

On the contrary, other studies did not confirm the association between early pregnancy loss and PCOS [315].

3.2.4.3 Gestational Diabetes

In normal pregnancy, maternal carbohydrate metabolism adapts to offer the fetus an adequate and continuous glucose supply despite intermittent maternal intake. The physiologic changes include pancreatic β-cell hyperplasia and an initial increase in insulin sensitivity followed by a progressive insulin resistance.

β-cell hyperplasia seems to be induced by prolactin and human placental lactogen; on the contrary, production of "diabetogenic hormones," such as GH and CRH, contributes to insulin resistance. This maternal insulin resistance, in turn, shunts nutrients to the fetus.

From the third trimester, fasting glucose concentrations are 10–20 % lower, postprandial glucose concentrations are significantly elevated and prolonged, and fasting insulin level is double that of nonpregnant women [216].

Thus, normal pregnancy induces a state of insulin resistance, and because women with PCOS have a high incidence of IR, they have an increased risk of developing gestational diabetic complications [316].

GDM is defined as carbohydrate intolerance that either begins in or is first recognized in pregnancy [317]. Its pathophysiology includes both insulin resistance and abnormalities of β-cell glucose sensitivity, which leads to inadequate insulin response [318].

According to a large study, PCOS women have a 2.4-fold increased odds of gestational diabetes, independent of age, race, and multiple gestation [319]. Furthermore, this increased risk occurs independent of obesity [320].

In fact, during the pregnancy, hyperinsulinemic women with PCOS develop more easily impaired glucose tolerance or gestational diabetes: the compensatory mechanism (reduced glucose clearance and/or defects of insulin action at receptor and post-receptor sites) that leads to prepregnancy hyperinsulinemia may more easily fail during pregnancy [321].

Investigators have shown that women with GDM with higher glucose values at OGTT, higher mean blood glucose, and worse glycemic control are at higher risk of preterm delivery [322].

Moreover, it was found that women with PCOS and GDM had a 3.5-fold higher risk for impaired glucose metabolism after delivery [323].

3.2.4.4 Pregnancy-Induced Hypertension

A meta-analysis showed that PCOS women have a higher risk of developing pregnancy-induced hypertension: this risk was also present after excluding all studies in which a higher BMI, multiple pregnancy rates, and a lower parity among women with PCOS were reported. Women with PCOS also demonstrated an increased incidence of preeclampsia of an order similar to that associated with multiple pregnancies. Moreover, older (age >30 years) women with PCOS are more susceptible to PIH than the younger women [324].

As widely explained in the previous chapter, hyperinsulinemia can cause endothelial dysfunction, and this association suggests a placental insufficiency in PCOS women [320], due to a vascular maladaptation: in fact, a study showed that arterial elasticity is impaired during the first trimester, while it decreases during the second and third trimester. It was also reported that systolic, diastolic, and mean arterial pressures were elevated throughout the pregnancy and that 27 % of the women with PCOS developed pregnancy-induced hypertension [325].

Furthermore, hyperandrogenemia in early second trimester and throughout pregnancy is associated with subsequent preeclampsia [326–330], and preeclampsia in a previous pregnancy is associated with elevated androgen levels later in life [330]. In fact, maternal androgen levels are higher in complicated compared to uncomplicated pregnancies in PCOS women [301]. This hypothesis was based on in vitro studies of preeclamptic placentas that were found to have decreased ability to aromatize androgens to estriol, compared to placentas from normal pregnancies [331].

3.2.4.5 Neonatal Outcome

Despite the risk of macrosomia due to the increased risk of gestational diabetes, the prevalence of SGA seems to be increased in PCOS women: 12.8 % vs 2.8 % of healthy controls, according to a Dutch study [332].

The cause can be found in the placental dysfunction or could be influenced by the mild raised number of preterm labor (1.75-fold higher risk).

Neonates of PCOS women have a 2.31 times higher risk of admission to intensive care unit and three times higher perinatal mortality than newborns of healthy women. Perinatal morbidity could be explained by prematurity and intrauterine growth retardation due to the placental dysfunction [333].

3.3   PCOS Phenotype in Different Ages

PCOS clinical and biochemical presentations and its metabolic consequences vary with age (Table 3.1) [334, 335].

3.3.1   Adolescence

The clinical presentation of chronic anovulation varies by age, with amenorrhea and oligomenorrhea being common among adolescents [336].

Menstrual irregularities and insulin resistance are common and usual features of normal puberty period, and they can make the diagnosis of PCOS in this period of life difficult [337].

Menstrual irregularity is common in the early years after menarche, and oligo-anovulation may be absolutely normal [338]: this is due to the immaturity of the hypothalamic–pituitary–ovarian (HPO) axis. An old study showed that 80 % of the cycles were anovulatory in the first year after menarche, 50 % in the third, and 10 % in the sixth: it is generally accepted that it may take up to 5 years after menarche for the HPO axis to reach maturation [339, 340].

The serum concentrations of sex hormones increase with age, from premenarchal to post-menarchal [339].

Table 3.1 PCOS features in different ages

Adolescence	Fertile period	Perimenopausal period
Chronic anovulation	Periods became more regular	Increased IGT, type II diabetes, hypertension, obesity, metabolic syndrome
Oligomenorrhea/amenorrhea	Increasing levels of insulin resistance	

Furthermore, concomitant eating disorders are frequent during these ages, and secondary amenorrhea can be associated with anorectic behavior in adolescents [341]. As ultrasound images have shown, uterine growth continues several years after menarche, and the average ovarian volume increases from early childhood until the age of 16 [342].

Regarding the ovarian morphology, the difference between a multifollicular appearance and polycystic ovarian morphology in adolescents is difficult to define [342]. About 80 % of girls have this USS finding and the presence of polycystic ovarian morphology in a non-hyperandrogenic adolescent should be considered normal [343].

Mild hair growth can be also considered a normal component of the late stages of puberty and early adolescence, because it can persist for several years; therefore, the diagnosis is often not made until later in life, when endocrine and metabolic dysfunctions have been firmly established [344].

In fact, the most important finding for clinical hyperandrogenism in female adolescents is progressive hirsutism [344]: acne and alopecia were not suggested as clinical markers for the diagnosis of PCOS in adolescents [345].

Premature pubarche, or the development of pubic and axillary hair before age 8 years, may be an early sign of PCOS [346]. Premature pubarche may occur as a result of some adrenal androgen disorders, but it could also be due to an idiopathic early activation of adrenal androgen secretion. However, not all girls with PCOS experience premature adrenarche; persistent hyperandrogenism remains a distinct feature of girls with premature pubarche who go on to develop PCOS, and the hyperandrogenism is exacerbated if a child develops obesity [347].

On the other hand, puberty period is normally associated with a mild insulin resistance: this is called "physiological peri-pubertal hyperinsulinemia," which together with increased GH levels is responsible for the "pubertal growth spurt"; the result is an accelerated bone, muscle, and adipose tissue growth.

Moreover, adolescent hyperandrogenemia is associated with a reduction in peripheral tissue insulin sensitivity and compensatory hyperinsulinemia, which implies an increase in the risk of type II diabetes [348]. The increased prevalence of obesity in the younger population leads to long-term consequences for cardiovascular disease at relatively young ages.

There is a strong inverse relationship between reported age and weight at menarche, suggesting that girls who were overweight had an earlier menarche, while those who were thin, compared with their peers, experienced a later menarche [349].

Earlier menarche in girls with PCOS might be expected based on findings that overweight girls experience earlier pubarche, thelarche, and menarche than those with a normal BMI [350, 351].

According to all these findings, a definitive diagnosis of PCOS in adolescents should require all three Rotterdam elements (not just 2 out of 3) [345].

3.3.2   Fertile Period

PCOS remains stable only during early adult age (18–30 years), but after that time, it changes in ovarian and adrenal function and in metabolic regulation modifying the presentation of the syndrome [352].

The menstrual cycles may become regular with age in women with PCOS [353, 354]: the development of a new balance in the polycystic ovary, caused merely by follicle loss through ovarian aging, can explain the occurrence of regular cycles in older patients with PCOS [354]. In a study of aging women with PCOS comparing those who became regular with those still menstruating irregularly, a lower follicle count for women with PCOS was predictive of the achievement of regular menstrual cycles with age [355], confirming that a decrease in the size of the follicle cohort from ovarian aging is largely responsible for the regular menstrual cycles in aging PCOS women [355]. The decrease in both ovarian volume and follicle number, caused by the aging, results in loss of PCO morphology [356].

The production of androgens in women may decrease because of ovarian aging or decreased production by the adrenal glands over time [357].

Normally, there is a marked decrease in adrenal androgen secretion, including androstenedione and DHEAS, between the ages of 40 and 45 years [358]; androgens levels also decline 20–30 % in women with PCOS.

A recent study, consisting in a 20-year follow-up of PCOS women, showed the inability to diagnose the disorder in about 10 % of women who had PCOS diagnosed 20 years earlier [359].

3.3.3   Premenopausal and Postmenopausal Period

Hyperandrogenism partially resolves before menopause in women with PCOS [360], but a recent study showed that adrenal androgen secretion also remains pronounced up to menopause in women with PCOS, indicating that exposure to hyperandrogenism persists for a long time in these women [361]: they have an elevated androgen to estrogen ratio.

It seems probable that long-lasting hyperandrogenism may magnify the unfavorable hormonal and metabolic changes related to menopause and expose these women to increased health risks [362].

Ovarian volume and follicle number decrease with age in women with and without PCOS [363].

AMH levels decreased with an increase in age in both the PCOS cases and normo-ovulatory controls [364]. AMH measurement could be useful in the prediction of the menopausal transition [365, 366]. Using AMH as a predictive marker, the reproductive lifespan of PCOS women is an average of 2 years longer than that of normo-ovulatory women [364].

Furthermore, aging may also be associated with a defect in insulin action [367]. In fact, age is an important risk factor for developing metabolic disorders and insulin resistance. Aging may also be associated with a defect in insulin action that is manifested by decreased whole-body tissue sensitivity to insulin without a change in tissue responsiveness [367]. The glucose intolerance may reflect part of the aging process. In elderly subjects, the severity of carbohydrate intolerance is directly correlated with the degree of peripheral insulin resistance [368].

A recent study has demonstrated that impaired glucose metabolism, enhanced ovarian androgen secretion, and chronic inflammation observed in premenopausal PCOS women persist after menopause [362].

As result, it is clearly noted that the most common symptoms in senior age are those related to metabolic syndrome.

Despite the longer exposure to cardiovascular risk factors, it is still difficult to demonstrate an increased risk of morbidity and mortality in women with PCOS: only two studies tried to study PCOS long-term outcomes, but no increased cardiovascular morbidity or raised risk of death, up to age 70 years, was pointed out [221, 369].

References

1. Rebar R, Judd HL, Yen SS et al (1976) Characterization of the inappropriate gonadotropin secretion in polycystic ovary syndrome. J Clin Invest 57:1320–1329
2. Hsueh AJW (1986) Paracrine mechanism involved in granulosa cell differentiation. Clin Endocrinol Metab 15:117–134
3. Erickson GF, Magoffin DA, Gabriel Garzo V et al (1992) Granulosa cells of polycystic ovaries: are they normal or abnormal? Hum Reprod 7:293–299
4. Mason HD, Willis DS, Beard RW et al (1994) Estradiol production by granulosa cells of normal and polycystic ovaries: relationship to menstrual cycle history and concentrations of gonadotropins and sex steroids in follicular fluid. J Clin Endocrinol Metab 79:1355–1360
5. Hillier SG (1994) Current concepts of the roles of follicle stimulating hormone and luteinizing hormone in folliculogenesis. Hum Reprod 9:188–191
6. Abbott DH, Dumesic DA, Franks S (2002) Developmental origin of polycystic ovary syndrome-hypothesis. J Endocrinol 174:1–5
7. Zawadzki JK, Dunaif A (1992) Diagnostic criteria for polycystic ovary syndrome; towards a rational approach. In: Dunaif A, Givens JR, Haseltine F, Merriam G (eds) Polycystic ovary syndrome. Blackwell Scientific, Boston, pp 377–384
8. Dunaif A (1997) Insulin resistance and the polycystic ovary syndrome: mechanism and implications for pathogenesis. Endocr Rev 18:774–800
9. Taylor AE, McCourt B, Martin KA et al (1997) Determinants of abnormal gonadotropin secretion in clinically defined women with polycystic ovary syndrome. J Clin Endocrinol Metab 82:2248–2256
10. Azziz R, Task Force on the Phenotype of the Polycystic Ovary Syndrome of the Androgen Excess PCOS Society et al (2009) The androgen excess and PCOS society criteria for the polycystic ovary syndrome: the complete task force report. Fertil Steril 91:456–488
11. Molli GW Jr, Rosenfield RL (1979) Testosterone binding and free plasma androgen concentrations under physiological conditions: characterization by flow dialysis technique. J Clin Endocrinol Metab 49:730–736

12. Nestler JE, Powers LP, Matt DW et al (1991) A direct effect of hyperinsulinemia on serum sex hormone-binding globulin levels in obese women with the polycystic ovary syndrome. J Clin Endocrinol Metab 72:83–89
13. Yildiz BO, Azziz R (2007) The adrenal and polycystic ovary syndrome. Rev Endocr Metab Disord 8:331–342
14. Lachelin GC, Barnett M, Hopper BR et al (1979) Adrenal function in normal women and women with the polycystic ovary syndrome. J Clin Endocrinol Metab 49:892–898
15. Billing H, Furuta I, Hsueh AJW (1993) Estrogens inhibit and androgen enhance ovarian granulosa cell apoptosis. Endocrinology 133:2204–2212
16. Okutsu Y et al (2010) Exogenous androstenedione induces formation of follicular cysts and premature luteinization of granulosa cells in the ovary. Fertil Steril 93:927–935
17. Ciotta L, Stracquadanio M et al (2011) Effects of Myo-inositol supplementation on oocyte's quality in PCOS patients: a double blind trial. Eur Rev Med Pharmacol Sci 15:509–514
18. DeVane GW, Czekala NM, Judd HL, Yen SS (1975) Circulating gonadotropins, estrogens, and androgens in polycystic ovarian disease. J Obstet Gynecol 121:496–500
19. Baird DT, Corker CS, Davidson DW et al (1977) Pituitary-ovarian relationships in polycystic ovary syndrome. J Clin Endocrinol Metab 45:798–801
20. MacDonald PC, Rombaut RP, Siiteri PK (1976) Plasma precursors of estrogen. Extent of conversion of plasma δ-4-androstenedione to estrone in normal males and nonpregnant normal, castrate and adrenalectomized females. J Clin Endocrinol Metab 27:1103–1111
21. Shen ZQ, Zhu HT, Lin JF (2008) Reverse of progestin-resistant atypical endometrial hyperplasia by metformin and oral contraceptives. Obstet Gynecol 112:465–467
22. Savaris RF, Groll JM, Young SL et al (2011) Progesterone resistance in PCOS endometrium: a microarray analysis in clomiphene citrate-treated and artificial menstrual cycles. J Clin Endocrinol Metab 96:1737–1746
23. Margarit L, Taylor A, Roberts MH et al (2010) MUC1 as a discriminator between endometrium from fertile and infertile patients with PCOS and endometriosis. J Clin Endocrinol Metab 95:5320–5329
24. Li X, Feng Y, Lin JF et al (2014) Endometrial progesterone resistance and PCOS. J Biomed Sci 21:2–8
25. Lee MM, Donahoe PK, Hasegawa T et al (1996) Mullerian inhibiting substance in humans: normal levels from infancy to adulthood. J Clin Endocrinol 81:571–576
26. Cook CL, Siow Y, Taylor S, Fallat M (2000) Serum mullerian inhibiting substance levels during normal menstrual cycles. Fertil Steril 73:859–861
27. Weenen C, Laven JS, Von Bergh AR et al (2004) Anti-mullerian hormone expression pattern in the human ovary: potential implications for initial and cyclic follicle recruitment. Mol Hum Reprod 10:77–83
28. Durlinger AL, Gruijters MJ, Kramer P et al (2002) Anti-mullerian hormone inhibits initiation of primordial follicle growth in the mouse ovary. Endocrinology 143:1076–1084
29. Durlinger AL, Visser JA, Themmen AP (2002) Regulation of ovarian function: the role of anti-mullerian hormone. Reproduction 124:601–609
30. Fallat ME, Siow Y, Marra M et al (1997) Mullerian inhibiting substance in follicular fluid and serum: a comparison of patients with tubal factor infertility, polycystic ovary syndrome and endometriosis. Fertil Steril 67:962–965
31. Cook C, Siow Y, Bremer AG, Fallat ME (2002) Relation between mullerian inhibiting substance and other reproductive hormones in untreated women with PCOS and normal women. Fertil Steril 77:141–146
32. Jonard S, Dewailly D (2004) The follicular excess in polycystic ovaries, due to ovarian hyperandrogenism, may be the culprit for the follicular arrest. Hum Reprod Update 10:107–117
33. Sahmay S, Aydin Y, Atakul N et al (2014) Relation of antimullerian hormone with the clinical signs of hyperandrogenism and polycystic ovary morphology. Gynecol Endocrinol 30(2):130–134
34. Pellat L, Rice S, Mason HD (2010) Anti-mullerian hormone and polycystic ovary syndrome: a mountain too high? Reproduction 139:825–833

35. Xi W, Gong F, Lu G (2012) Correlation of serum anti-mullerian hormone concentrations on day 3 of the in vitro fertilization stimulation cycle with assisted reproduction outcome in polycystic ovary syndrome patients. J Assist Reprod Genet 29:397–402

36. Piouka A, Farmakiotis D, Katsikis I et al (2009) Anti-mullerian hormone levels reflect severity of PCOS but are negatively influenced by obesity: relationship with increased luteinizing hormone levels. Am J Physiol Endocrinol Metab 296:E238–E243

37. Febregues F, Castelo-Branco C, Carmona F et al (2011) The effect of different hormone therapies on anti-mullerian hormone serum levels in anovulatory women of reproductive age. Gynecol Endocrinol 27:216–224

38. Dewailly D, Pigny P, Soudan B et al (2010) Reconciling the definitions of polycystic ovary syndrome: the ovarian follicle number and serum anti-mullerian hormone concentrations aggregate with the markers of hyperandrogenism. J Clin Endocrinol Metab 95: 4399–4405

39. Caglar GS, Kayaouglu I, Pabuccu R et al (2013) Anti-mullerian hormone and insulin resistance in classic phenotype lean PCOS. Arch Gynecol Obstet 288:905–910

40. Rojas J, Chavez M, Olivar L et al (2014) Polycystic ovary syndrome, insulin resistance, and obesity: navigating the pathophysiologic labyrinth. Int J Reprod Med. http://dx.doi.org/10.1155/2014/719050

41. Brassard M, AinMelk Y, Baillargeon JP (2008) Basic infertility including polycystic ovary syndrome. Med Clin North Am 92:1163–1192

42. Brower M, Brennan K, Pall M, Azziz R (2013) The severity of menstrual dysfunction as a predictor of insulin resistance in PCOS. J Clin Endocrinol Metab 98(12):E1967–E1971

43. Strowitzki T, Capp E, von Eye CH (2010) The degree of cycle irregularity correlates with the grade of endocrine and metabolic disorders in PCOS patients. Eur J Obstet Gynecol Reprod Biol 149:178–181

44. Chittenden BG, Fullerton G, Maheswari A, Bhattacharya S (2009) Polycystic ovary syndrome and the risk of gynaecological cancer: a systematic review. Reprod Biomed Online 19:398–405

45. Hardiman P, Pillay OC, Atiomo W (2003) Polycystic ovary syndrome and endometrial carcinoma. Lancet 361:1810–1812

46. Teede H, Deeks A, Moran L (2010) Polycystic ovary syndrome: a complex condition with psychological, reproductive and metabolic manifestations that impacts on health across the lifespan. BMC Med 8(41):1741–7015

47. Chakraborty P, Goswami SK, Rajani S et al (2013) Recurrent pregnancy loss in polycystic ovary syndrome: role of hyperhomocysteinemia and insulin resistance. PLoS One 8:e64446

48. Kalra S et al (2013) Is the fertile window extended in women with polycystic ovary syndrome? Utilizing the society for assisted reproductive technology registry to assess the impact of reproductive aging on live-birth rate. Fertil Steril 100:208–213

49. Redmond GP, Bergfeld WF (1990) Diagnostic approach to androgen disorders in women: acne, hirsutism, and alopecia. Cleve Clin J Med 57:423–427

50. Uno H (1986) Biology of hair growth. Semin Reprod Endocrinol 4:131–141

51. Wendelin DS, Pope DN, Mallory SB (2003) Hypertrichosis. J Am Acad Dermatol 48:161–179

52. Al-Nuaimi Y, Baier G, Watson REB et al (2010) The cycling hair follicle as an ideal systems biology research model. Exp Dermatol 19:707–713

53. Burger HG (2002) Androgen production in women. Fertil Steril 77:S3–S5

54. Alonso L, Fuchs E (2006) The hair cycle. J Cell Sci 119(Pt3):391–393

55. Escobar-Morreale HF, Carmina E, Dewailly D et al (2012) Epidemiology, diagnosis and management of hirsutism: a consensus statement by the androgen excess and polycystic ovary syndrome society. Hum Reprod Update 18:146–170

56. Zouboulis CC (2004) Acne and sebaceous gland function. Clin Dermatol 22:360–366

57. Zouboulis CC, Degitz K (2004) Androgen action on human skin—from basic research to clinical significance. Exp Dermatol 13(supplement 4):5–10

58. Makrantonaki E, Ganceviciene R, Zouboulis C (2011) An update on the role of the sebaceous gland in the pathogenesis of acne. Derm Endocrinol 3:41–49

59. Cela E, Robertson C, Rush K et al (2003) Prevalence of polycystic ovaries in women with androgenic alopecia. Eur J Endocrinol 149:439–442
60. Price VH (2003) Androgenetic alopecia in women. J Invest Dermatol Symp Proc 8:24–27
61. Daniel CR III, Iorizzo M, Piraccini BM, Tosti A (2011) Simple onycholysis. Cutis 87:226–228
62. Van de Kerkhof PCM, Paschc MC, Scher RK et al (2005) Brittle nail syndrome: a pathogenesis-based approach with a proposed grading system. J Am Acad Dermatol 53:644–651
63. Femiano F, Rullo R, Serpico R et al (2009) An unusual case of oral hirsutism in a patient with polycystic ovarian syndrome. Oral Med Oral Pathol Oral Radiol Endod 108:e13–e16
64. Canaris GJ, Manowitz NR, Mayor G et al (2000) The Colorado thyroid disease prevalence study. Arch Intern Med 160:526–534
65. Dayan CM, Daniels GH (1996) Chronic autoimmune thyroiditis. N Engl J Med 335:99–107
66. Cooper DS (2001) Subclinical hypothyroidism. N Engl J Med 345:260–265
67. Petrikova J, Lazurova I, Yehuda S (2010) Polycystic ovary syndrome and autoimmunity. Eur J Intern Med 21:369–371
68. Benetti-Pinto CL, Santana Berini Piccolo VR, Garmes HM et al (2013) Subclinical hypothyroidism in young women with polycystic ovary syndrome: an analysis of clinical, hormonal, and metabolic parameters. Fertil Steril 99(2):588–592
69. Mueller A, Schofl C, Dittrich R et al (2009) Thyroid stimulating hormone is associated with insulin resistance independently of body mass index and age in women with polycystic ovary syndrome. Hum Reprod 24:2924–2930
70. Kelley DE, Mandarino LJ (1988) Fuel selection in human skeletal muscle in insulin resistance: a reexamination. Diabetes 49:677–683
71. Kelley DE, Goodpaster B, Wing RR, Simoneau JA (1999) Skeletal muscle fatty acid metabolism in association with insulin resistance, obesity and weight loss. Am J Physiol 277:E1130–E1141
72. Ukropcova B, Sereda O, de Jonge L et al (2007) Family history of diabetes links impaired substrate switching and reduced mitochondrial content in skeletal muscle. Diabetes 56:720–727
73. Diamanti-Kandaris E, Dunaif A (2012) Insulin resistance and the polycystic ovary syndrome revisited: an update on mechanisms and implications. Endocr Rev 33:981–1030
74. Glueck CJ, Papanna R, Wang P et al (2003) Incidence and treatment of metabolic syndrome in newly referred women with confirmed polycystic ovarian syndrome. Metabolism 52:908–915
75. Ehrmann DA et al (2006) Prevalence and predictors of metabolic syndrome in women with polycystic ovary syndrome. J Clin Endocrinol Metab 91:48–53
76. Apridonidze et al (2005) Prevalence and characteristics of the metabolic syndrome in women with polycystic ovary syndrome. J Clin Endocrinol Metab 90:1929–1935
77. Ford ES et al (2002) Prevalence of the metabolic syndrome among US adults: findings from the third National Health and Nutrition Examination Survey. JAMA 287:356–359
78. Hoffman LK, Ehrmann DA (2008) Cardiometabolic features of polycystic ovary syndrome. Nat Clin Pract Endocrinol Metab 4(4):215–222
79. Coviello AD, Legro RS, Dunaif A (2006) Adolescent girls with polycystic ovary syndrome have an increased risk of the metabolic syndrome associated with increasing androgen levels independent of obesity and insulin resistance. J Clin Endocrinol Metab 91:492–497
80. Leibel NI, Baumann E, Kocherginsky M, Rosenfield R (2006) Relationship of adolescent polycystic ovary syndrome to parental metabolic syndrome. J Clin Endocrinol Metab 91:1275–1283
81. Haffner S, Taegtmeyer H (2003) Epidemic obesity and metabolic syndrome. Circulation 108(13):1541–1545
82. Dunaif A, Finegood DT (2006) Beta-cell dysfunction independent of obesity and glucose intolerance in the polycystic ovary syndrome. J Clin Endocrinol Metab 81:942–947
83. Ehrmann DA, Sturis J, Byrne MM et al (1995) Insulin secretory defects in polycystic ovary syndrome. Relationship to insulin sensitivity and family history of non-insulin-dependent diabetes mellitus. J Clin Invest 96:520–527

84. Mahabeer S, Jialal I, Norman RJ et al (1989) Insulin and C-peptide secretion in non-obese patients with polycystic ovarian disease. Horm Metab Res 21:502–506
85. O'Meara NM, Blackman JD, Ehrmann DA et al (1993) Defects in beta-cell function in functional ovarian hyperandrogenism. J Clin Endocrinol Metab 76:1241–1247
86. Cara JF et al (1998) Insulin-like growth factor I and insulin potentiate luteinizing hormone-induced androgen synthesis by rat ovarian thecal-interstitial cells. Endocrinology 123:733–739
87. Dunaif A et al (1989) Profound peripheral insulin resistance, independent of obesity, in polycystic ovary syndrome. Diabetes 38:1165–1174
88. Lambrinoudaki I (2010) Cardiovascular risk in postmenopausal women with the polycystic ovary syndrome. Maturitas 68(1):13–16
89. Mohamed-Ali V, Pinkney JH, Coppack SW (1998) Adipose tissue as an endocrine and paracrine organ. Int J Obes Relat Metab Disord 22:1145–1158
90. Spiegelman BM, Flier JS (1996) Adipogenesis and obesity: rounding out the big picture. Cell 87:377–389
91. Fruhbeck G (2004) The adipose tissue as a source of vasoactive factors. Curr Med Chem Cardiovasc Hematol Agents 2:197–208
92. Lee YH, Pratley RE (2005) The evolving role of inflammation in obesity and metabolic syndrome. Curr Diab Rep 5(1):70–75
93. Hausman DB, DiGirolamo M, Bartness TJ et al (2001) The biology of white adipocyte proliferation. Obes Rev 2(4):239–254
94. Weisberg SP, McCann D, Desai M et al (2003) Obesity is associated with macrophage accumulation in adipose tissue. J Clin Invest 112:1796–1808
95. Kershaw EE, Flier JS (2004) Adipose tissue as an endocrine organ. J Clin Endocrinol Metab 89:2548–2556
96. Rondinone CM (2006) Adipocyte-derived hormones, cytokines, and mediators. Endocrine 29:81–90
97. Yu YH, Ginsberg HN (2005) Adipocyte signaling and lipid homeostasis: sequelae of insulin-resistant adipose tissue. Circ Res 96:1042–1052
98. Halleux CM, Takahashi M, Delporte ML et al (2001) Secretion of adiponectin and regulation of apM1 gene expression in human visceral adipose tissue. Biochem Biophys Res Commun 288:1102–1107
99. Matsubara M, Maruoka S, Katayose S (2002) Decreased plasma adiponectin concentrations in women with dyslipidemia. J Clin Endocrinol Metab 87:2764–2769
100. Yang WS, Lee WJ, Funahashi T, Tanaka S et al (2001) Weight reduction increases plasma levels of an adipose-derived anti-inflammatory protein, adiponectin. J Clin Endocrinol Metab 86:3815–3819
101. Kazumi T, Kawaguchi A, Yoshino G et al (2002) Young men with high-normal blood pressure have lower serum adiponectin, smaller LDL size, and higher elevated heart rate than those with optimal blood pressure. Diabetes Care 25:971–976
102. Weyer C, Funahashi T, Tanaka S et al (2001) Hypoadiponectinemia in obesity and type 2 diabetes: close association with insulin resistance and hyperinsulinemia. J Clin Endocrinol Metab 86:1930–1935
103. Stefan N, Bunt JC, Salbe AD et al (2002) Plasma adiponectin concentrations in children: relationships with obesity and insulinemia. J Clin Endocrinol Metab 87:4652–4656
104. Arita Y, Kihara S, Ouchi N et al (1999) Paradoxical decrease of an adipose-specific protein, adiponectin, in obesity. Biochem Biophys Res Commun 257:79–83
105. Hotta K, Funahashi T, Arita Y et al (2000) Plasma concentrations of a novel, adipose-specific protein, adiponectin, in type 2 diabetic patients. Arterioscler Thromb Vasc Biol 20:1595–1599
106. Spranger J, Kroke A et al (2003) Adiponectin and protection against type 2 diabetes mellitus. Lancet 361:226–228
107. Toulis KA, Goulis DG et al (2009) Adiponectin levels in women with polycystic ovary syndrome: a systematic review and a meta-analysis. Hum Reprod Update 15:297–307

108. Barber TM, Franks S (2013) Adipocyte biology in polycystic ovary syndrome. Mol Cell Endocrinol 373:68–76

109. Fruhbeck G, Gomez-Ambrosi J (2001) Modulation of the leptin-induced white adipose tissue lipolysis by nitric oxide. Cell Signal 13:827–833

110. Maffei M, Halaas J, Ravussin E et al (1995) Leptin levels in human and rodent: measurement of plasma leptin and obRNA in obese and weight-reduced subjects. Nat Med 1:1155–1161

111. Calvar CE, Intebi AD, Bengolea SV et al (2003) Leptin in patients with polycystic ovary syndrome. Direct correlation with insulin resistance. Medicina (B Aires) 63:704–710

112. Zachow RJ, Magoffin DA (1997) Direct intraovarian effects of leptin: impairment of the synergistic action of insulin-like growth factor-I on follicle-stimulating hormone-dependent estradiol-17 beta production by rat ovarian granulosa cells. Endocrinology 138:847–850

113. Wang P, Vanhoutte PM, Miao CY (2011) Visfatin and cardio-cerebro-vascular disease. J Cardiovasc Pharmacol 59:1–9

114. Yildiz BO, Bozdag G, Otegen U et al (2010) Visfatin and retinol-binding protein 4 concentrations in lean, glucose-tolerant women with PCOS. Reprod Biomed Online 20:150–155

115. Cekmez F, Cekmez Y, Pirgon O et al (2011) Evaluation of new adipocytokines and insulin resistance in adolescents with polycystic ovary syndrome. Eur Cytokine Netw 22:32–37

116. Dikmen E, Tarkun I, Canturk Z, Cetinarslan B (2010) Plasma visfatin level in women with polycystic ovary syndrome. Gynecol Endocrinol 27:475–479

117. Manneras-Holm L, Leonhardt H, Kullberg J et al (2011) Adipose tissue has aberrant morphology and function in PCOS: enlarged adipocytes and low serum adiponectin, but not circulating sex steroids, are strongly associated with insulin resistance. J Clin Endocrinol Metab 96:E304–E311

118. Villa J, Pratley RE (2011) Adipose tissue dysfunction in polycystic ovary syndrome. Curr Diab Rep 11:179–184

119. Faulds G, Ryden M, Wahrenberg H, Arner P (2003) Mechanisms behind lipolytic catecholamine resistance of subcutaneous fat cells in the polycystic ovary syndrome. J Clin Endocrinol Metab 88:2269–2273

120. Dicker A, Ryden M, Naslund E et al (2004) Effect of testosterone on lipolysis in human preadipocytes from different fat depots. Diabetologia 47:420–428

121. Dunaif A, Segal KR, Shelley DR et al (1992) Evidence for distinctive and intrinsic defects in insulin action in polycystic ovary syndrome. Diabetes 41:1257–1266

122. Ciaraldi TP, Morales AJ, Hickman MG et al (1997) Cellular insulin resistance in adipocytes from obese polycystic ovary syndrome subjects involves adenosine modulation of insulin sensitivity. J Clin Endocrinol Metab 82:1421–1425

123. Diamanti-Kandarakis E, Papavassiliou AG (2006) Molecular mechanisms of insulin resistance in polycystic ovary syndrome. Trends Mol Med 12:324–332

124. Danforth JE (2000) Failure of adipocyte differentiation causes type II diabetes mellitus? Nat Genet 26(1):13

125. Barber TM, McCarthy MI, Wass JA, Franks S (2006) Obesity and polycystic ovary syndrome. Clin Endocrinol (Oxf) 65:137–145

126. Giagulli VA, Verdonck L, Giorgino R, Vermeulen A (1989) Precursors of plasma androstanediol-and androgen-glucuronides in women. J Steroid Biochem 33:935–940

127. Stewart PM, Shackleton CH, Beastall GH, Edwards CR (1990) 5 alpha-reductase activity in polycystic ovary syndrome. Lancet 355:431–433

128. Fassnacht M, Schlenz N, Schneider SB et al (2003) Beyond adrenal and ovarian androgen generation: increased peripheral 5alpha-reductase activity in women with polycystic ovary syndrome. J Clin Endocrinol Metab 88:2760–2766

129. Tsilchorozidou T, Honour JW, Conway GS (2003) Altered cortisol metabolism in polycystic ovary syndrome: insulin enhances 5alpha-reduction but not the elevated adrenal steroid production rates. J Clin Endocrinol Metab 88:5907–5913

130. Chin D, Shackleton C, Prasad VK et al (2000) Increased 5alpha-reductase and normal 11 beta-hydroxysteroid dehydrogenase metabolism of C19 and C21 steroids in a young population with polycystic ovarian syndrome. J Pediatr Endocrinol Metab 13:253–259

131. Engeli S, Schling P, Gorzelniak K et al (2003) The adipose tissue renin-angiotensin-aldosterone system: role in the metabolic syndrome. Int J Biochem Cell Biol 35:807–825
132. Lee YH, Nair S, Rousseau E et al (2005) Microarray profiling of isolated abdominal subcutaneous adipocytes from obese vs non-obese Pima Indians: increased expression of inflammation-related genes. Diabetologia 48(9):1776–1783
133. Nonogaki K, Fuller GM, Fuentes NL et al (1995) Interleukin-6 stimulates hepatic triglyceride secretion in rats. Endocrinology 136:2143–2149
134. Kelly CC, Lyall H, Petrie JR et al (2001) Low grade chronic inflammation in women with polycystic ovarian syndrome. J Clin Endocrinol Metab 86:2453–2455
135. Bahceci M, Tuzcu A, Canoruc N et al (2004) Serum C-reactive protein (CRP) levels and insulin resistance in non-obese women with polycystic ovarian syndrome, and effect of bicalutamide on hirsutism, CRP levels and insulin resistance. Horm Res 62:283–287
136. Meden-Vrtovec H, Vrtovec B, Osredkar J (2007) Metabolic and cardiovascular changes in women with polycystic ovary syndrome. Int J Gynecol Obstet 99:87–90
137. Cho LW, Randeva HS, Atkin SL (2007) Cardiometabolic aspects of polycystic ovarian syndrome. Vasc Health Risk Manag 3(1):55–63
138. Hahn S, Haselhorst U, Tan S et al (2006) Low serum 25-hydroxyvitamin D concentrations are associated with insulin resistance and obesity in women with polycystic ovary syndrome. Exp Clin Endocrinol Diabetes 114:577–583
139. Holick MF (2007) Vitamin D deficiency. N Engl J Med 357:266–281
140. Pittas AG, Lau J, Hu FB, Dawson-Hughes B (2007) The role of vitamin D and calcium in type 2 diabetes. A systematic review and meta-analysis. J Clin Endocrinol Metab 92:2017–2029
141. Freundlich M, Quiroz Y, Zhang Z et al (2008) Suppression of renin-angiotensin gene expression in the kidney by paricalcitol. Kidney Int 74:1394–1402
142. Chiu KC, Chu A, Go VL, Saad MF (2004) Hypovitaminosis D is associated with insulin resistance and beta cell dysfunction. Am J Clin Nutr 79:820–825
143. Isaia G, Giorgino R, Adami S (2001) High prevalence of hypovitaminosis D in female type 2 diabetic population. Diabetes Care 24:1496
144. Bikle D (2009) Nonclassic actions of vitamin D. J Clin Endocrinol Metabol 94:26–34
145. Shoelson SE, Herrero L, Naaz A (2007) Obesity, inflammation, and insulin resistance. Gastroenterology 132:2169–2180
146. Wehr E, Pilz S et al (2009) Association of hypovitaminosis D with metabolic disturbances in polycystic ovary syndrome. Eur J Endocrinol 161:575–582
147. Glintborg D, Andersen M, Hagen C, Hermann AP (2005) Higher bone mineral density in Caucasian, hirsute patients of reproductive age. Positive correlation of testosterone levels with bone mineral density in hirsutism. Clin Endocrinol (Oxf) 62:683–691
148. Balen AH, Conway GS, Kaltsas G et al (1995) Polycystic ovary syndrome: the spectrum of the disorder in 1741 patients. Hum Reprod 10:2107–2111
149. Carmina E, Koyama T, Chang L et al (1992) Does ethnicity influence the prevalence of adrenal hyperandrogenism and insulin resistance in polycystic ovary syndrome? Am J Obstet Gynecol 167:1807–1812
150. Silfen ME, Denburg MR, Manibo AM et al (2003) Early endocrine, metabolic, and sonographic characteristics of polycystic ovary syndrome (PCOS): comparison between nonobese and obese adolescents. J Clin Endocrinol Metab 88:4682–4688
151. Norman RJ, Wu R, Stankiewicz MT (2004) Polycystic ovary syndrome. Med J Aust 180:132–137
152. Bjorntrop P (1997) Obesity. Lancet 350:423–426
153. Basdevant A, Raison J, Guy-Grand B (1987) Influence of the distribution of the body fat on vascular risk. Presse Med 16:167–170
154. Lefebvre P, Bringer J, Renard E et al (1997) Influence of weight, body fat patterning and nutrition on the management of PCOS. Hum Reprod 12(Suppl 1):72–81
155. Kirchengast S et al (2001) Body composition characteristics and body fat distribution in lean women with polycystic ovary syndrome. Hum Reprod 16:1255–1260

156. Horejsi R et al (2004) Android subcutaneous adipose tissue topography in lean and obese women suffering from PCOS: comparison with type 2 diabetic women. Am J Phys Anthropol 124:275–281

157. Svendsen P, Nilas L, Norgaard K et al (2008) Obesity, body composition and metabolic disturbances in polycystic ovary syndrome. Hum Reprod 23:2113–2121

158. Williams DP, Boyden TW, Pamenter RW et al (1993) Relationship of body fat percentage and fat distribution with DHEA-S in premenopausal females. J Clin Endocrinol Metab 77:80–85

159. Douchi T, Ijuin H, Nakamura S et al (1995) Body fat distribution in women with polycystic ovary syndrome. Obstet Gynecol 86:516–519

160. Arner P (2005) Human fat cell lipolysis: biochemistry, regulation and clinical role. Best Pract Res Clin Endocrinol Metab 19:471–482

161. Nesto R (2004) C-reactive protein, its role in inflammation, type 2 diabetes and cardiovascular disease and the effects of insulin-sensitising treatment with thiazolidinediones. Diabetes Med 21:810–817

162. Bays H, Mandarino L, DeFronzo RA (2004) Role of the adipocyte, free fatty acids and ectopic fat in the pathogenesis of type 2 diabetes mellitus: a peroxisome proliferators-activated· receptor agonists provide a rational therapeutic approach. J Clin Endocrinol Metab 89:463–478

163. Hsuch WA, Lyon CJ, Quinones MJ (2004) Insulin resistance and the endothelium. Am J Med 117:109–117

164. Bhattacharya SM (2010) Insulin resistance and overweight-obese women with polycystic ovary syndrome. Gynecol Endocrinol 26(5):344–347

165. Masuzaki H, Flier JS (2003) Tissue-specific glucocorticoid reactivating enzyme, 11-beta-hydroxysteroid dehydrogenase type 1 – a promising drug target for the treatment of metabolic syndrome. Curr Drug Targets Immune Endocr Metab Disord 3:255–262

166. Legro RS et al (1998) Evidence for a genetic basis for hyperandrogenemia in polycystic ovary syndrome. Proc Natl Acad Sci U S A 95:14956–14960

167. Third report of the National Cholesterol education Program (NCEP) (2002) Expert panel on detection, evaluation, and treatment of high blood cholesterol in adults (Adult Treatment Panel III) final report. Circulation 106:3143–3421

168. Wild R (2012) Dyslipidemia in PCOS. Steroids 77:295–299

169. Pirwany IR, Fleming R et al (2001) Lipids and lipoprotein subfractions in women with PCOS: relationship to metabolic and endocrine parameters. Clin Endocrinol (Oxf) 54(4):447–453

170. Pekala P, Kawakami M, Vine W et al (1983) Studies of insulin resistance in adipocytes induced by macrophage mediator. J Exp Med 157:1360–1365

171. Wild RA, Alaupovic P, Parker IJ (1992) Lipid and apolipoprotein abnormalities in hirsute women. I. The association with insulin resistance. Am J Obstet Gynecol 166(4):1191–1196

172. Ginsberg HN, Brown WV (2011) Apolipoprotein CIII: 42 years old and even more interesting. Arterioscler Thromb Vasc Biol 31(3):471–473

173. Dietschy JM, Brown MS (1974) Effect of alterations of the specific activity of the intracellular acetyl CoA pool on apparent rates of hepatic cholesterogenesis. J Lipid Res 15:508–516

174. Cupisti S, Giltay EJ, Gooren LJ et al (2010) The impact of testosterone administration to female-to-male transsexuals on insulin resistance and lipid parameters compared with women with polycystic ovary syndrome. Fertil Steril 94:2647–2653

175. Fruzzetti F, Perini D, Lazzarini V et al (2009) Adolescent girls with polycystic ovary syndrome showing different phenotypes have a different metabolic profile associated with increasing androgen levels. Fertil Steril 92:626–634

176. Diamanti-Kandarakis E, Papavassiliou AG, Kandarakis SA et al (2007) Pathophysiology and types of dyslipidemia in PCOS. Trends Endocrinol Metab 18:280–285

177. Legro RS (2001) Prevalence and predictors of dyslipidemia in women with polycystic ovary syndrome. Am J Med 111:607–613

178. Conway GS, Agrawal R, Betteridge DJ et al (1992) Risk factors for coronary artery disease in lean and obese women with the polycystic ovary syndrome. Clin Endocrinol (Oxf) 37:119–125

179. Holte J, Bergh T, Berne C et al (1994) Serum lipoprotein lipid profile in women with the polycystic ovary syndrome: relation to anthropometric, endocrine and metabolic variables. Clin Endocrinol (Oxf) 41:463–471

180. Legro RS, Blanche P, Krauss RM et al (1999) Alterations in low-density lipoprotein and high-density lipoprotein subclasses among Hispanic women with polycystic ovary syndrome: influence of insulin and genetic factors. Fertil Steril 72:990–995

181. Robinson S, Henderson AD, Gelding SV et al (1996) Dyslipidaemia is associated with insulin resistance in women with polycystic ovaries. Clin Endocrinol (Oxf) 44:277–284

182. Wild RA, Painter PC, Coulson PB et al (1985) Lipoprotein lipid concentrations and cardiovascular risk in women with polycystic ovary syndrome. J Clin Endocrinol Metab 61:946–951

183. Rocha MP, Marcondes JAM, Barcellos CRG et al (2011) Dyslipidemia in women with polycystic ovary syndrome: incidence, pattern and predictors. Gynecol Endocrinol 27(10):814–819

184. Wilson PW, Abbott RD, Castelli WP (1988) High density lipoprotein cholesterol and mortality. The Framingham heart study. Arteriosclerosis 8:737–741

185. Vrbikova J, Zamrazilova H, Sedlackova B, Snajderova M (2011) Metabolic syndrome in adolescents with polycystic ovary syndrome. Gynecol Endocrinol 27(10):820–822

186. Cohen JC, Horton JD, Hobbs HH (2011) Human fatty liver disease: old questions and new insights. Science 332:1519–1523

187. Ciotta L, Pagano I, Stracquadanio M, Formuso C (2011) Incidenza di sindrome dell'ovaio policistico in giovani donne affette da steatosi epatica non alcolica. Minerva Ginecol 63:429–437

188. Ahima RS (2007) Insulin resistance: cause or consequence of nonalcoholic steatohepatitis? Gastroenterology 132:444–446

189. Clark JM, Brancati FL, Diehl AM (2003) The prevalence and etiology of elevated aminotransferase levels in the United States. Am J Gastroenterol 98:960–967

190. Cortez-Pinto H, de Moura MC, Day CP (2006) Non-alcoholic steatohepatitis: from cell biology to clinical practice. J Hepatol 44:197–208

191. Schwimmer JB, Khorram O, Chiu V, Schwimmer WB (2005) Abnormal aminotransferase activity in women with polycystic ovary syndrome. Fertil Steril 83:494–497

192. Setji TL, Holland ND, Sanders LL et al (2006) Nonalcoholic steatohepatitis and nonalcoholic fatty liver disease in young women with polycystic ovary syndrome. J Clin Endocrinol Metab 91:1741–1747

193. Lavine JE, Schwimmer JB (2004) Nonalcoholic fatty liver disease in the pediatric population. Clin Liver Dis 8:549

194. Cerda C, Perez-Ayuso RM et al (2007) Nonalcoholic fatty liver disease in women with polycystic ovary syndrome. J Hepatol 47:412–417

195. Gambarin-Gelwan M, Kinkhabwala SV, Schiano TD et al (2007) Prevalence of nonalcoholic fatty liver disease in women with polycystic ovary syndrome. Clin Gastroenterol Hepatol 5:496–501

196. Baranova A, Tran TP, Birerdinc A, Younossi ZM (2011) Systematic review: association of polycystic ovary syndrome with metabolic syndrome and non-alcoholic fatty liver disease. Aliment Pharmacol Ther 33:801–814

197. Jones H, Sprung V, Pugh CJA et al (2012) Polycystic ovary syndrome with hyperandrogenism is characterized by an increased risk of hepatic steatosis compared to nonhyperandrogenic PCOS phenotypes and healthy controls, independent of obesity and insulin resistance. J Clin Endocrinol Metab 97(10):3709–3716

198. Brzozowska MM, Ostapowicz G, Weltman MD (2009) An association between non-alcoholic fatty liver disease and polycystic ovarian syndrome. J Gastroenterol Hepatol 24:243–247

199. Barfield E, Liu YH, Kessler M et al (2009) The prevalence of abnormal liver enzymes and metabolic syndrome in obese adolescent females with polycystic ovary syndrome. J Pediatr Adolesc Gynecol 22:318–322
200. Cascella T, Palomba S et al (2006) Serum aldosterone concentration and cardiovascular risk in women with polycystic ovarian syndrome. J Clin Endocrinol Metab 91:4395–4400
201. Zavaroni I, Coruzzi P, Bonini L et al (1995) Association between salt sensitivity and insulin concentrations in patients with hypertension. Am J Hypertens 8:855–858
202. Resnick LM (1992) Cellular calcium and magnesium metabolism in the pathophysiology and treatment of hypertension and related metabolic disorders. Am J Med 93:11S–20S
203. Muller-Wieland D, Kotzka J, Knebel et al (1998) Metabolic syndrome and hypertension: pathophysiology and molecular basis of insulin resistance. Basic Res Cardiol 93(Suppl 2): 131–134
204. Sechi LA, Bartoli E (1996) Molecular mechanisms of insulin resistance in arterial hypertension. Blood Press Suppl 1:47–54
205. Reaven GM, Lithell H, Landsberg L (1996) Hypertension and associated metabolic abnormalities – the role of insulin resistance and the sympathoadrenal system. N Engl J Med 334:374–381
206. Barcellos CRG, Rocha MP, Hayashida SAY et al (2007) Impact of body mass index on blood pressure levels in patients with polycystic ovary syndrome. Arq Bras Endocrinol Metab 51(7):1104–1109
207. Orio F Jr et al (2004) The cardiovascular risk of young women with polycystic ovary syndrome: an observational, analytical, prospective case-control study. J Clin Endocrinol Metab 89:3696–3701
208. Yarali H et al (2001) Diastolic dysfunction and increased serum homocysteine concentrations may contribute to increased cardiovascular risk in patients with polycystic ovary syndrome. Fertil Steril 76:511–516
209. Dahlgren E et al (1992) Women with polycystic ovary syndrome wedge resected in 1956 to 1965: a long-term follow-up focusing on natural history and circulating hormones. Fertil Steril 57:507–513
210. Zimmerman S et al (1992) Polycystic ovary syndrome: lack of hypertension despite profound insulin resistance. J Clin Endocrinol Metab 75:508–513
211. Dahlgren E et al (1992) Polycystic ovary syndrome and risk of myocardial infarction: evaluated from a risk factor model based on a prospective population study of women. Acta Obstet Gynecol Scand 71:599–604
212. Holte J et al (1996) Elevated ambulatory day-time blood pressure in women with polycystic ovary syndrome: a sign of pre-hypertensive state? Hum Reprod 11:23–28
213. Elting MW, Korsen TJM, Bezemer PD et al (2001) Prevalence of diabetes mellitus, hypertension and cardiac complaints in a follow-up study of a Dutch PCOS population. Hum Reprod 16:556–660
214. Cibula D, Cifkova R, Fanta M et al (2000) Increased risk of non-insulin dependent diabetes mellitus, arterial hypertension and coronary artery disease in perimenopausal women with a history of the polycystic ovary syndrome. Hum Reprod 15:785–789
215. Vrbikova J, Cifkova R et al (2003) Cardiovascular risk factors in young Czech females with polycystic ovary syndrome. Hum Reprod 18:980–984
216. Pauli JM, Raja-Khan N, Wu X, Legro RS (2011) Current perspectives of insulin resistance and polycystic ovary syndrome. Diabet Med 28(12):1445–1454
217. Ehrmann DA, Barnes RB, Rosenfield RL et al (1999) Prevalence of impaired glucose tolerance and diabetes in women with polycystic ovary syndrome. Diabetes Care 22:141–146
218. Celik C, Tasdemir N, Abali R et al (2014) Progression to impaired glucose tolerance or type 2 diabetes mellitus in polycystic ovary syndrome: a controlled follow-up study. Fertil Steril 101:1123–1128
219. Kim JJ, Choi YM, Cho YM et al (2012) Prevalence of elevated glycated hemoglobin in women with polycystic ovary syndrome. Hum Reprod 27:1439–1444

220. Barrett-Connor E, Giardina EG, Gitt AK et al (2004) Women and heart disease: the role of diabetes and hyperglycemia. Arch Intern Med 164(9):934–942
221. Wild S, Pierpoint T, McKeigue P, Jacobs H (2000) Cardiovascular disease in women with polycystic ovary syndrome at long-term follow-up: a retrospective cohort study. Clin Endocrinol (Oxf) 52:595–600
222. Bierwolf C, Struve K, Marshall L et al (1997) Slow wave sleep drives inhibition of pituitary-adrenal secretion in humans. J Neuroendocrinol 9:479–484
223. Ip MS, Lam B, Ng MM et al (2002) Obstructive sleep apnea is independently associated with insulin resistance. Am J Respir Crit Care Med 165:670–676
224. Punjabi NM, Sorkin JD, Katzel LI et al (2002) Sleep-disordered breathing and insulin resistance in middle-aged and overweight men. Am J Respir Crit Care Med 165:677–682
225. Meslier N, Gagnadoux F, Giraud P et al (2003) Impaired glucose-insulin metabolism in males with obstructive sleep apnoea syndrome. Eur Respir J 22:156–160
226. Punjabi NM, Shahar E, Redline S et al (2004) Sleep-disordered breathing, glucose intolerance, and insulin resistance: the sleep heart health study. Am J Epidemiol 160:521–530
227. Tassone F, Lanfranco F, Gianotti L et al (2003) Obstructive sleep apnoea syndrome impairs insulin sensitivity independently of anthropometric variables. Clin Endocrinol (Oxf) 59:374–379
228. Rexrode KM et al (2003) Sex hormone levels and risk of cardiovascular events in postmenopausal women. Circulation 108:1688–1693
229. Vgontzas AN et al (2001) Polycystic ovary syndrome is associated with obstructive sleep apnea and daytime sleepiness: role of insulin resistance. J Clin Endocrinol Metab 86:517–520
230. Fogel RB et al (2001) Increased prevalence of obstructive sleep apnea syndrome in patients with polycystic ovarian syndrome. J Clin Endocrinol Metab 86:1175–1180
231. Gopal M et al (2002) The role of obesity in the increased prevalence of obstructive sleep apnea syndrome in patients with polycystic ovarian syndrome. Sleep Med 3:401–404
232. Mokhlesi B, Scoccia B, Mazzone T, Sam S (2012) Risk of obstructive sleep apnea in obese and non-obese women with polycystic ovary syndrome and healthy reproductively normal women. Fertil Steril 97(3):786–791
233. Tasali E, Van Cauter E, Ehrmann DA (2006) Relationships between sleep disordered breathing and glucose metabolism in polycystic ovary syndrome. J Clin Endocrinol Metab 91:36–42
234. Tasali E, Van Cauter E, Hoffman L, Ehrmann DA (2008) Impact of obstructive sleep apnea on insulin resistance and glucose tolerance in women with polycystic ovary syndrome. J Clin Endocrinol Metab 93:3878–3884
235. Driver HS, McLean H, Kumar DV et al (2005) The influence of the menstrual cycle on upper airway resistance and breathing during sleep. Sleep 28:449–456
236. Pien GW, Schwab RJ (2004) Sleep disorders during pregnancy. Sleep 27:1405–1417
237. Popovic RM, White DP (1998) Upper airway muscle activity in normal women: influence of hormonal status. J Appl Physiol 84:1055–1062
238. Randeva H, Tan BK et al (2012) Cardiometabolic aspects of the polycystic ovary syndrome. Endocr Rev 33(5):812–841
239. Bauer K (1993) Laboratory markers of coagulation activation. Arch Pathol Lab Med 117:71–77
240. Lowe GDO (1987) Blood rheology in general medicine and surgery. Baillieres Clin Haematol 1:827–862
241. Mchedlishvili G (1998) Disturbed blood flow structuring as critical factor of hemorheological disorders in microcirculation. Clin Hemorheol Microcirc 19:315–325
242. Patterson W, Caldwell C, Doll D (1990) Hyperviscosity syndromes and coagulopathies. Semin Oncol 17:210–216
243. Koenig W, Sund M et al (1998) Plasma viscosity and the risk of coronary heart disease: results from the MONICA-Augsburg Cohort Study, 1984 to 1992. Arterioscler Thromb Vasc Biol 18:768–772

244. Koenig W, Sund M et al (2000) Association between plasma viscosity and all-cause mortality: results from the MONICA-Augsburg Cohort Study 1984–92. Br J Haematol 109:453–458

245. Coata G, Ventura F, Lombardini R et al (1995) Effect of low-dose oral triphasic contraceptives on blood viscosity, coagulation and lipid metabolism. Contraception 52:151–157

246. Erdem NT, Ercan M et al (2003) Plasma viscosity as an early cardiovascular risk factor in hirsute women with eumenorrhea or oligomenorrhea. Fertil Steril 80:1195–2008

247. Vervita V, Saltamavros AD, Adonakis G et al (2009) Obesity and insulin resistance increase plasma viscosity in young women with polycystic ovary syndrome. Gynecol Endocrinol 25(10):640–646

248. Caimi G, Sinagra D, Scarpitta AM, Lo Presti R (2001) Plasma viscosity and insulin resistance in metabolic syndrome. Int J Obestet 25:1856–1857

249. Ercan M, Konukoglu D (2008) Role of plasma viscosity and plasma homocysteine level on hyperinsulinemic obese female subjects. Clin Hemorheol Microcirc 38:227–234

250. Sola E, Vaya A, Simo M et al (2007) Fibrinogen, plasma viscosity and blood viscosity in obesity. Relationship with insulin resistance. Clin Hemorheol Microcirc 37:309–318

251. Dereli D, Ozgen G, Buyukkececi F et al (2003) Platelet dysfunction in lean women with polycystic ovary syndrome and association with insulin sensitivity. J Clin Endocrinol Metab 88:2263–2268

252. Trovati M, Mularoni EM, Burzacca S et al (1995) Impaired insulin-induced platelet antiaggregating effect in obesity and in obese NIDDM patients. Diabetes 44:1318–1322

253. Ruggeri ZM (2002) Platelets in atherothrombosis. Nat Med 8:1227–1234

254. Gawaz M, Neumann FJ, Dickfeld T et al (1997) Vitronectin receptor (alpha(v)beta3) mediates platelet adhesion to the luminal aspect of endothelial cells: implications for reperfusion in acute myocardial infarction. Circulation 96:1809–1818

255. Gawaz M, Brand K, Dickfeld T et al (2000) Platelets induce alterations of chemotactic and adhesive properties of endothelial cells mediated through an interleukin-1-dependent mechanism. Implications for atherogenesis. Atherosclerosis 148:75–85

256. Tateson JE, Moncada S, Jr V (1977) Effects of prostacyclin (Pgx) on cyclic AMP concentrations in human platelets. Prostaglandins 13:389–397

257. Shimokawa H (1999) Primary endothelial dysfunction: atherosclerosis. J Mol Cell Cardiol 31:23–37

258. Orio JRF, Palomba S, Cascella T et al (2004) Early impairment of endothelial structure and function in young normal-weight women with polycystic ovary syndrome. J Clin Endocrinol Metab 89:4588–4593

259. Kelly CJG, Speirs A, Gould GW et al (2002) Altered vascular function in young women with polycystic ovary syndrome. J Clin Endocrinol Metab 87:742–746

260. Vincent D, Ilany J, Kondo T et al (2003) The role of endothelial insulin signalling in the regulation of vascular tone and insulin resistance. J Clin Invest 111:1372–1380

261. Vryonidou A, Papatheodorou A, Tavridou A et al (2005) Association of hyperandrogenemic and metabolic phenotype with carotid intima-media thickness in young women with polycystic ovary syndrome. J Clin Endocrinol Metab 90:2740–2746

262. Paradisi G, Steinberg HO, Hempfling A et al (2001) Polycystic ovary syndrome is associated with endothelial dysfunction. Circulation 103:1410–1415

263. Bickerton AS, Clark N, Meeking D et al (2005) Cardiovascular risk in women with polycystic ovarian syndrome (PCOS). J Clin Pathol 58:151–154

264. Kawashima S, Yokoyama M (2004) Dysfunction of endothelial nitric oxide synthase and atherosclerosis. Arterioscler Thromb Vasc Biol 24:998–1005

265. Bitar MS, Wahid S, Mustafa S et al (2005) Nitric oxide dynamics and endothelial dysfunction in type II model of genetic diabetes. Eur J Pharmacol 511:53–64

266. Bhagat K, Vallance P (1999) Effects of cytokines on nitric oxide pathways in human vasculature. Curr Opin Nephrol Hypertens 8:89–96

267. Chan WPA, Ngo DT, Sverdlov AL et al (2013) Premature aging of cardiovascular/platelet function in polycystic ovary syndrome. Am J Med 126:640.e1–640.e7

268. Ouchi N, Ohishi M, Kihara S et al (2003) Association of hypoadiponectinemia with impaired vasoreactivity. Am J Med 42:231–234
269. Tan KC, Xu A, Chow WS et al (2004) Hypoadiponectinemia is associated with impaired vasoreactivity. J Clin Endocrinol Metab 89:765–769
270. Motoshima H, Wu X, Mahadev K, Goldstein BJ (2003) Adiponectin suppresses proliferation and superoxide generation and enhances NOS activity in endothelial cells treated with oxidized LDL. Biochem Biophys Res Commun 315:264–271
271. Fernandez-Real JM, Castro A, Vazquez G et al (2004) Adiponectin is associated with vascular function independent of insulin sensitivity. Diabetes Care 27:739–745
272. Matsuda M, Shimomura I, Sata M et al (2002) Role of adiponectin in preventing vascular stenosis: the missing link of adipovascular axis. Biol Chem 277:27487–37491
273. Okamoto Y, Kihara S, Ouchi N et al (2002) Adiponectin reduces atherosclerosis in apolipoprotein E-deficient mice. Circulation 106:2767–2770
274. Gonzalez F, Rote NS, Minium J, Kirwan JP (2006) Increased activation of nuclear factor kB triggers inflammation and insulin resistance in polycystic ovary syndrome. J Clin Endocrinol Metab 91:1508–1512
275. Piotrowski PC, Rzepczynska IJ et al (2005) Oxidative stress induces expression of CYP11A, CYP17, STAR and 3bHSD in rat theca-interstitial cells. J Soc Gynecol Investig 12(2 Suppl):319 A
276. Escobar-Morreale HF, Luque-Ramírez M, González F (2011) Serum inflammatory markers in polycystic ovary syndrome: a systematic review and meta-analysis. Fertil Steril 95:1048–1058
277. Blake G, Ridker P (2001) Novel clinical markers of vascular wall inflammation. Circ Res 89:763–771
278. Engin-Ustun Y, Ustun Y et al (2006) Are polycystic ovaries associated with cardiovascular disease risk as polycystic ovary syndrome. Gynecol Endocrinol 22(6):324–328
279. Yeh ET, Willerson JT (2003) Coming of age of C-reactive protein: using inflammation markers in cardiology. Circulation 107:370–371
280. Talbott EO et al (2004) The relationship between C-reactive protein and carotid intima-media thickness in middle-aged women with polycystic ovary syndrome. J Clin Endocrinol Metab 89:6061–6067
281. Talbottt EO et al (2004) Evidence for an association between metabolic cardiovascular syndrome and coronary and aortic calcification among women with polycystic ovary syndrome. J Clin Endocrinol Metab 89:5454–5461
282. Christian RC et al (2003) Prevalence and predictors of coronary artery calcification in women with polycystic ovary syndrome. J Clin Endocrinol Metab 88:2562–2568
283. Shroff R et al (2007) Young obese women with polycystic ovary syndrome have evidence of early coronary atherosclerosis. J Clin Endocrinol Metab 92:4609–4614
284. Vanky E, Stridskelv S, Skogoy K et al (2011) PCOS – what matters in early pregnancy? Data from a cross-sectional, multicenter study. Acta Obstet Gynecol Scand 90:398–404
285. Freeman EW et al (2007) Association of anti-mullerian hormone levels with obesity in late reproductive-age women. Fertil Steril 87:101–106
286. Santoro N et al (2004) Body size and ethnicity are associated with menstrual cycle alterations in women in the early menopausal transition: the Study of Women's Health across the Nation (SWAN) Daily Hormone Study. J Clin Endocrinol Metab 89:2622–2631
287. Robker RL et al (2009) Obese women exhibit differences in ovarian metabolites, hormones, and gene expression compared with moderate-weight women. J Clin Endocrinol Metab 94:1533–1540
288. Cardozo E, Pavone ME, Hirshfeld-Cytron JE (2011) Metabolic syndrome and oocyte quality. Trends Endocrinol Metab 22:103–109
289. Agarwal A et al (2005) Role of oxidative stress in female reproduction. Reprod Biol Endocrinol 3:28
290. Marquard KL et al (2010) Polycystic ovary syndrome and maternal obesity affect oocyte size in in vitro fertilization/intracytoplasmic sperm injection cycles. Fertil Steril. doi:10.1016/j.fertnstert.2010.10.026

291. Chakraborty P, Goswami SK, Rajani S et al (2013) Recurrent pregnancy loss in polycystic ovary syndrome: role of hyperhomocysteinemia and insulin resistance. PLoS One 8(e64446):1–6

292. Rai R, Clifford K, Regan L (1996) The modern preventative treatment of recurrent miscarriage. Br J Obstet Gynaecol 103:106–110

293. Rai R, Backos M, Rushworth F, Regan I (2000) Polycystic ovaries and recurrent miscarriage – a reappraisal. Hum Reprod 15:612–615

294. Amer SAK, Gopalan V, Li TC et al (2002) Long term follow-up of patients with polycystic ovarian syndrome after laparoscopic ovarian drilling: clinical outcome. Hum Reprod 17:2035–2042

295. Ford HB, Schust DJ (2009) Recurrent pregnancy lost: etiology, diagnosis and therapy. Rev Obstet Gynecol 2:76–83

296. Jacubowics DJ, Iuorno MJ et al (2002) Effects of metformin on early pregnancy loss in the polycystic ovary syndrome. J Clin Endocrinol Metab 87(2):524–529

297. Jacobs HS, Homburg RR (1990) The endocrinology of conception. Baillieres Clin Endocrinol Metab 4:195–205

298. Van der Spuy ZM, Dyer SJ (2004) The pathogenesis of infertility and early pregnancy loss in polycystic ovary syndrome. Best Pract Res Clin Obstet Gynecol 18:755–771

299. Fenkci V, Fenkci S et al (2003) Decreased total antioxidant status and increased oxidative stress in women with polycystic ovary syndrome may contribute to the risk of cardiovascular disease. Fertil Steril 80:123–127

300. Diamanti-Kandarakis E, Paterakis T et al (2006) Indices of low-grade chronic inflammation in polycystic ovary syndrome and the beneficial effect of metformin. Hum Reprod 21:1426–1431

301. Vanky E, Salvesen KA, Asberg A, Carlsen SM (2008) Haemoglobin, C-reactive protein and androgen levels in uncomplicated and complicated pregnancies of women with polycystic ovary syndrome. Scand J Clin Lab Invest 68:421–426

302. Palomba S, Russo T, Falbo A et al (2012) Decidual endovascular trophoblast invasion in women with polycystic ovary syndrome: an experimental case-control study. J Clin Endocrinol Metab 97:2441–2449

303. Giudice LC (2006) Endometrium in PCOS: implantation and predisposition to endocrine CA. Best Pract Res Clin Endocrinol Metab 20:235–244

304. Tian L, Shen H, Lu Q et al (2007) Insulin resistance increases the risk of spontaneous abortion after assisted reproduction technology treatment. J Clin Endocrinol Metab 92:1430–1433

305. Maryam K, Bouzari Z, Basirat Z et al (2012) The comparison of insulin resistance frequency in patients with recurrent early pregnancy loss to normal individuals. BMC Res Notes 5:133. doi:10.1186/1756-0500-5-133

306. Sun L, Lv H, Wei W et al (2010) Angiotensin-converting enzyme D/I and plasminogen activator inhibitor-1 4G/5G gene polymorphisms are associated with increased risk of spontaneous abortions in polycystic ovarian syndrome. J Endocrinol Invest 33:77–82

307. Gosman GG, Katcher HI, Legro RS (2006) Obesity and the role of gut and adipose hormones in female reproduction. Hum Reprod Update 12:585–601

308. Atiomo WU, Bates SA, Condon JE et al (1998) The plasminogen activator inhibitor system in women with polycystic ovary syndrome. Fertil Steril 69:236–241

309. Schacter M, Raziel A, Friedler S et al (2003) Insulin resistance in patients with polycystic ovary syndrome is associated with elevated plasma homocysteine. Hum Reprod 18:721–727

310. Wijeyaratne CN, Nirantharakumar K, Balen AH et al (2004) Plasma homocysteine in polycystic ovary syndrome: does it correlate with insulin resistance and ethnicity? Clin Endocrinol 60:560–567

311. Boxmeer JC, Steegers-Theunissen R, Lindemans J et al (2008) Homocysteine metabolism in the pre-ovulatory follicle during ovarian stimulation. Hum Reprod 23:2570–2576

312. Ebisch IM, Peters WH, Thomas CM et al (2006) Homocysteine, glutathione and related thiols affect fertility parameters in the (sub) fertile couple. Hum Reprod 21:1725–1733

313. Nafiye Y, Sevtap K, Muammer D et al (2010) The effect of serum and intrafollicular insulin resistance parameters and homocysteine levels of non-obese, nonhyperandrogenemic polycystic ovary syndrome patients on in vitro fertilization outcome. Fertil Steril 93:1864–1869
314. Motta AB (2012) The role of obesity in the development of polycystic ovary syndrome. Curr Pharm Des 18:2482–2491
315. Tulppala M, Stenman UH, Cacciatore B, Ylikorkala O (1993) Polycystic ovaries and levels of gonadotrophins and androgens in recurrent miscarriage: prospective study in 50 women. Br J Obstet Gynaecol 100:348–352
316. Legro RS, Castracane VD, Kauffman RP (2004) Detecting insulin resistance in polycystic ovary syndrome: purposes and pitfalls. Obstet Gynecol Surv 59:141–154
317. American College of Obstetricians and Gynecologists (ACOG) (2001) Gestational diabetes. ACOG Practice Bulletin, n. 30. Obstet Gynecol 98:525–538
318. Catalano PM, Kirwan JP, Haugel-de Mouzon S, King J (2003) Gestational diabetes and insulin resistance: role in short and long-term implications for mother and fetus. J Nutr 133:1674S–1683S
319. Lo JC, Feigenbaum SL, Escobar GJ et al (2006) Increased prevalence of gestational diabetes mellitus among women with diagnosed polycystic ovary syndrome: a population-based study. Diabetes Care 29:1915–1917
320. Boomsma CM, Eijkemans MJCE, Hughes EG et al (2006) A meta-analysis of pregnancy outcomes in women with polycystic ovary syndrome. Hum Reprod Update 12:673–683
321. Lanzone A, Fulghesu AM, Cucinelli F et al (1996) Preconceptional and gestational evaluation of insulin secretion in patients with polycystic ovary syndrome. Hum Reprod 11:2382–2386
322. Yogev Y, Langer O (2007) Spontaneous preterm delivery and gestational diabetes: the impact of glycemic control. Arch Gynecol Obstet 276:361–365
323. Palomba S, Falbo A, Russo T et al (2012) The risk of a persistent glucose metabolism impairment after gestational diabetes mellitus is increased in patients with polycystic ovary syndrome. Diabetes Care 35:861–867
324. Haakova L, Cibula D, Rezabek K et al (2003) Pregnancy outcome in women with PCOS and in controls matched by age and weight. Hum Reprod 18:1438–1441
325. Hu S, Leonard A, Seifalian A, Hardiman P (2007) Vascular dysfunction during pregnancy in women with polycystic ovary syndrome. Hum Reprod 22:1532–1539
326. Carlsen SM, Romundstad P, Jacobsen G (2004) Early second trimester hyperandrogenemia and subsequent preeclampsia: a prospective study. Acta Obstet Gynecol Scand 84:117–121
327. Serin IS, Kula M, Basbug M et al (2001) Androgen levels of preeclamptic patients in the third trimester of pregnancy and six weeks after delivery. Acta Obstet Gynecol Scand 80:1009–1013
328. Steier JA, Ulstein M, Myking OL (2002) Human chorionic gonadotropin and testosterone in normal and preeclamptic pregnancies in relation to fetal sex. Obstet Gynecol 100:552–556
329. Troisi R, Potischman N, Roberts JM et al (2003) Maternal serum oestrogen and androgen concentrations in preeclamptic and uncomplicated pregnancies. Int J Epidemiol 32:455–460
330. Laivuori H, Kaaja R, Rutanen EM et al (1998) Evidence of high circulating testosterone in women with prior preeclampsia. J Clin Endocrinol Metab 83:344–347
331. Hahnel ME, Martin JD, Michael CA, Hahnel R (1989) Metabolism of androstenedione by placental microsomes in pregnancy hypertension. Clin Chim Acta 181:103–108
332. Homburg R (2006) Pregnancy complications in PCOS. Best Pract Res Clin Endocrinol Metab 20:281–292
333. Boomsma CM, Fauser BC, Macklon NS (2008) Pregnancy complications in women with polycystic ovary syndrome. Semin Reprod Med 26(1):72–84
334. Pasquali R, Gambineri A (2006) Polycystic ovary syndrome: a multifaceted disease from adolescence to adult age. Ann N Y Acad Sci 1092:158–174
335. Rodriguez-Moran M, Guerrero-Romero F (2003) Insulin resistance is independently related to age in Mexican women. J Endocrinol Invest 26:42–48

336. Mansfield MJ, Emans SJ (1984) Adolescent menstrual irregularity. J Reprod Med 29:399–410
337. Diamanti-Kandarakis E (2010) PCOS in adolescents. Best Pract Res Clin Obstet Gynaecol 24:173–183
338. Apter D, Vihko R (1985) Premenarcheal endocrine changes in relation to age at menarche. Clin Endocrinol (Oxf) 22:160–753
339. Apter D (1980) Serum steroids and pituitary hormones in female puberty: a partly longitudinal study. Clin Endocrinol (Oxf) 12:107–120
340. Hsu M-I (2013) Changes in the PCOS phenotype with age. Steroids 78:761–766
341. Wiksten-Almstromer M, Hirschberg AL, Hagenfeldt K (2008) Prospective follow-up of menstrual disorders in adolescence and prognostic factors. Acta Obstet Gynecol Scand 87:1162–1168
342. Holm K, Laursen EM, Brocks V, Muller J (1995) Pubertal maturation of the internal genitalia: an ultrasound evaluation of 166 healthy girls. Ultrasound Obstet Gynecol 6:175–181
343. Codner E, Villarroel C, Eyzaguirre FC et al (2011) Polycystic ovarian morphology in postmenarchal adolescents. Fertil Steril 95:702–706
344. Jeffrey CR, Coffler MS (2007) Polycystic ovary syndrome: early detection in the adolescent. Clin Obstet Gynecol 50:178–187
345. Carmina E, Oberfield SE, Lobo RA (2010) The diagnosis of polycystic ovary syndrome in adolescents. Am J Obstet Gynecol 203:201.e1–201.e5
346. Ibanez L, Potau N, Virdis R et al (1993) Postpubertal outcome in girls diagnosed of premature pubarche during childhood: increased frequency of functional ovarian hyperandrogenism. J Clin Endocrinol Metab 76:1599–1603
347. McCartney CR, Blank SK, Prendergast KA et al (2007) Obesity and sex steroid changes across puberty: evidence for marked hyperandrogenemia in pre- and early pubertal obese girls. J Clin Endocrinol Metab 92:430–436
348. Lewy VD, Danadian K, Witchel SF, Arslanian S (2001) Early metabolic abnormalities in adolescent girls with polycystic ovary syndrome. J Pediatr 138:38–44
349. Carroll J, Saxena R, Welt CK (2012) Environmental and genetic factors influence age at menarche in women with polycystic ovary syndrome. J Pediatr Endocrinol Metab 25:459–466
350. Rosenfield RL, Lipton RB, Drum ML (2009) Thelarche, pubarche, and menarche attainment in children with normal and elevated body mass index. Pediatrics 123:84–88
351. Stark O, Peckham CS, Moynihan C (1989) Weight and age at menarche. Arch Dis Child 64:383–387
352. Welt CK, Carmina E (2013) Lifecycle of polycystic ovary syndrome (PCOS): from in utero to menopause. J Clin Endocrinol Metab 98(12):4629–4638
353. Birdsall MA, Farquhar CM (1996) Polycystic ovaries in pre and post-menopausal women. Clin Endocrinol (Oxf) 44:269–276
354. Elting MW, Korsen TJ, Rekers-Mombarg LT, Schoemaker J (2000) Women with polycystic ovary syndrome gain regular menstrual cycles when ageing. Hum Reprod 15:24–28
355. Elting MW, Kwee J, Korsen TJ et al (2003) Aging women with polycystic ovary syndrome who achieve regular menstrual cycles have a smaller follicle cohort than those who continue to have irregular cycles. Fertil Steril 79:1154–1160
356. Rotterdam ESHRE/ASRM-Sponsored PCOS Consensus Workshop Group (2004) Revised 2003 consensus on diagnostic criteria and long-term health risks related to polycystic ovary syndrome (PCOS). Hum Reprod 19:41–47
357. Brown ZA, Louwers YV, Fong SL et al (2011) The phenotype of polycystic ovary syndrome ameliorates with aging. Fertil Steril 96:1259–1265
358. Davison SL, Bell R, Donath S et al (2005) Androgen levels in adult females: changes with age, menopause and oophorectomy. J Clin Endocrinol Metab 90:3847–3853
359. Carmina E, Campagna AM, Lobo RA (2012) A 20-year follow-up of young women with polycystic ovary syndrome. Obstet Gynecol 119:263–269
360. Winters SJ, Talbott E, Guzick DS et al (2000) Serum testosterone level decrease in middle age in women with polycystic ovary syndrome. Fertil Steril 73:724–729

361. Puurunen J, Piltonen T, Jaakola P et al (2009) Adrenal androgen production capacity remains high up to menopause in women with polycystic ovary syndrome. J Clin Endocrinol Metab 94:1973–1978
362. Puurunen J, Piltonen T, Morin-Papunen L et al (2011) Unfavorable hormonal, metabolic, and inflammatory alterations persist after menopause in women with PCOS. J Clin Endocrinol Metab 96(6):1827–1834
363. Alsamarai S, Adams JM, Murphy MK et al (2009) Criteria for polycystic ovarian morphology in polycystic ovary syndrome as a function of age. J Clin Endocrinol Metab 94:4961–4970
364. Tehrani FR, Solaymani-Dodaran M, Hedayati M, Azizi F (2010) Is polycystic ovary syndrome an exception for reproductive aging? Hum Reprod 25:1775–1781
365. La Marca A, Volpe A (2006) Anti-mullerian hormone (AMH) in female reproduction: is measurement of circulating AMH a useful tool? Clin Endocrinol (Oxf) 64:603–610
366. Lambalk CB, van Disseldorp J, de Koning CH, Broekmans FJ (2009) Testing ovarian reserve to predict age at menopause. Maturitas 63:280–291
367. Rowe JW, Minaker KL, Pallotta JA, Flier SJ (1983) Characterization of the insulin resistance of aging. J Clin Invest 71:1581–1587
368. Fink RI, Kolterman OG, Griffin J, Olefsky JM (1983) Mechanisms of insulin resistance in aging. J Clin Invest 71:1523–1535
369. Schmidt J, Landin-Wilhelmsen K et al (2011) Cardiovascular disease and risk factors in PCOS women of postmenopausal age: a 21-year controlled follow-up study. J Clin Endocrinol Metab 96:3794–3803

Psychological Implications of PCOS

4

Agata Ando' and Antonio Maria D'Alessandro

Nowadays, quality of life (QoL) is widely considered an important parameter for evaluating the quality and outcome of health care, particularly for patients suffering from chronic disorders: polycystic ovary syndrome is one of these.

Clinical symptoms of PCOS could compromise women's quality of life and have a strong negative effect on mood, psychological well-being, and sexual satisfaction.

Physically visible PCOS symptoms are more likely to provoke distress in younger women than older women [1].

The "American College of Obstetricians and Gynecologists" suggests that, in view of the high prevalence rate of depression and persistence of new cases in PCOS population, an initial evaluation of all PCOS women should also include assessment of mental health disorders.

The PRIME-MD PMQ (Primary Care Evaluation of Mental Disorders Patient Health Questionnaire) [2] is suitable to evaluate eating disorders [3]; furthermore, its interpretation and scoring are very simple.

4.1 PCOS Symptoms and Psychological Correlation

4.1.1 Obesity and Body Image

Dissatisfaction with body image is one of the major causes for psychological disorders even in a healthy population; most women affected by PCOS are overweight, and having a high BMI exposes them to several appearance-related challenges.

Some studies showed that PCOS women have lower quality of life and overweight was the largest contributor to poor QoL [4]. In fact, health-related quality of life questionnaires in women with PCOS have shown that excess weight and difficulties with losing weight are the foremost concerns [5].

Moreover, by using PCOSQ (Health-Related Quality of Life Questionnaire for Women with Polycystic Ovary Syndrome), it was demonstrated that higher levels

© Springer International Publishing Switzerland 2015
M. Stracquadanio, L. Ciotta, *Metabolic Aspects of PCOS: Treatment with Insulin Sensitizers*, DOI 10.1007/978-3-319-16760-2_4

of BMI related with lower scores (reported by respondent), which is indicative of several weight-related concerns [6].

Personal negative judgments regarding own body appear to be associated with the difficulty to begin close and romantic relationships.

Women with PCOS report that they are not happy with the way they look or the way that clothes fit them and consequently do not feel their body is sexually appealing [8]: these feelings are negatively associated with self-esteem, body satisfaction, and fear of negative appearance evaluation [9].

In fact, a poor body representation in PCOS women may be conditioned by cultural influences as it has been shown that android fat pattern, commonly associated with PCOS, is considered unattractive in many cultures [10, 11].

4.1.2 Hirsutism

Women with PCOS recognize excessive hair growth (especially on face) as the second most severe symptom negatively affecting on their life satisfaction [12].

Some women, in fact, describe themselves using masculine terms such as "beard" or "mustache," and they are frustrated because they look at their bodies as a failure of their femininity [13, 14].

The presence of facial hair is one of the most essential and visible differences between men and women: hair on a female face reflects a symbolic transgression between the two genders [15].

As shown in a qualitative study, hirsute women feel "slaves of their own body" and describe this condition as a "prison" [16]. Moreover, looking in the mirror very often could represent an obsessive-compulsive behavior [17].

4.1.3 Infertility and Sexual Life

Characteristic symptoms of PCOS occur during a life period in which relationships, marriage, and having a child play an important role: for this reason, changes in femininity are likely to mean an increased risk of psychological distress [7].

As any cause of infertility, even PCOS could lead to exaggerated emotional states depending on lots of variables such as period of time spent in trying to conceive and number of attempted therapies.

Several factors predicting the impact of PCOS-associated infertility upon HRQoL (health-related quality of life) have been identified: PCOS women who had been pregnant but had miscarriage experience reported the lowest scores on the infertility field, exceeding those who had been unsuccessful in having pregnancy [6].

Some patients are infertile and are subjected to social pressure due to the importance given to having children by the society.

Having a partner who supports the hope of having a child was found to be a protective factor and improves the emotional well-being of PCOS patients [18].

Moreover, according to a study, even adolescent girls with PCOS are 3.4 times more likely than healthy girls to be "worried about their ability to become pregnant in the future" compared to the controls; however, this fear was not associated with odds of having sexual intercourse [19, 20].

Menstrual irregularities are associated to low feminine identity too [13]. Oligo-/amenorrhea can have important social consequences, especially in many Muslim backgrounds. For example, the tenets of Islam decree that menstruating women are not allowed to pray [20]. If a woman prays every day, without the expected monthly stop of 4–5 days, her social entourage will be aware that she is experiencing menstrual irregularities [21].

PCOS has also a negative effect on sexual functioning, even when data are adjusted for BMI; the main reason is the low self-esteem and constant concerns about their appearance. Based on the study of Elsenbruch et al. "women with PCOS did not differ from others in the frequency of their sexual activity and sexual thoughts; they were less satisfied with their sexual life and found themselves less attractive thinking that their partners find them less attractive and remain sexually unsatisfied while being with them" [7].

Moreover, in another study a substantial portion of women with PCOS reported that they most often took the initiative to have sexual intercourse in the relationship [22, 23]. Could this be related to the increased testosterone levels in PCOS women? No associations were found. An alternative psychological explanation is that some women with PCOS felt that their partners were not attracted by them [7].

4.2 PCOS and Mental Disorders

4.2.1 Mood Disorders

Mood disorders include major depressive disorder (MDD), dysthymic disorder, and depression not otherwise specified based on DSM-IV [24].

In healthy people, depression can cause or exacerbate clinical symptoms such as fatigue, poor sleep, and changes in appetite and weight. In those with chronic illness, depression can have more insidious consequences, influencing the expression and course of disease [25].

Several studies have been investigating the association between PCOS and depression. The result is that PCOS women reported more depressive symptoms compared with the control group [7, 26] and scored above average on questionnaires assessing depression [27, 28].

The prevalence of depression in women with PCOS is high, ranging from 28 to 64 % [29–31]. Studies found that 14 % of women suffering from PCOS reported suicidal ideation. This percentage is high as what has been reported from other chronic medical conditions and much higher than in the general population [32].

Despite this, there are discordant opinions about the real cause: neither androgenization nor excessive hair growth showed significant correlation with depression [27]. In fact, it was not observed any significant differences in total or free testosterone levels or in the adrenal androgen DHEAS between depressed women with PCOS and non-depressed women with PCOS [33].

Two-thirds of women with PCOS show weight problems, but it is not properly correlated only to PCOS: in fact, high BMI might increase depression in the normal population as well [34–36].

Some studies found depressed women with PCOS to have a higher evidence of insulin resistance and impaired fasting glucose than PCOS women without depression [27, 33].

There are plausible physiological connections between depression and insulin resistance; in fact, depression has been associated with increased cortisol, amplified sympathetic activity, decreased central nervous system serotonin, and increased inflammatory markers: these features are also associated with insulin resistance [37].

Depression is also associated with behaviors that worsen insulin resistance, including unhealthy eating and physical inactivity. These findings may explain why depression predisposes to diabetes [38].

In view of all these data and because the peak incidence of depression is during the reproductive years, gynecologists have to be able to identify and treat women with PCOS who have depression.

4.2.2 Anxiety

According to the DSM-IV, diagnostic criteria for GAD (generalized anxiety disorder) include excessive anxiety and apprehension about events or activities, occurring more days than not, for at least 6 months; abnormal anxiety becomes a problem when it occurs without any recognizable motivation or when the stimulus does not warrant that kind of reaction [39].

Anxiety symptoms could be identified in one-third of PCOS patients, especially social phobia [32, 35, 40]. It has been associated mainly with hirsutism [17], acne [41], obesity [42], and infertility [43].

The prevalence of anxiety in women with PCOS ranges from 34 to 57 % [31, 44].

Fears reported by hirsute women are mainly categorized as "social phobia" or anxiety-evoking situations, such as meeting strangers, attending parties, shopping, and mixing at work [6].

PCOS women with higher anxiety scores showed significantly elevated insulin resistance and FAI (free androgen index) values than PCOS with lower anxiety score, independently out of BMI [45].

Some authors have suggested that adolescents with PCOS are at higher risk for anxiety symptoms related to the clinical signs of hyperandrogenism. In a study of hirsute 13–18-year-old girls, anxiety was diagnosed in 26 % compared with 10 % in the control girls [46]. Furthermore, successful treatment of hirsutism leads to a reduction of time spent on hair removal with a consequent improvement in anxiety score [47].

The risk of developing coexistent depression and anxiety in women with PCOS is unknown [39]. An interesting study found that 15 % of PCOS patients had coexistent anxiety and depression. Coexisting anxiety in depressed patients may worsen the outcome increasing the risk of suicide, worsening overall symptoms, conferring a poorer response to treatment, increasing the number of medically unexplained symptoms, and increasing functional disability [48].

Most women with PCOS reported sleep disorders: a partial explanation for this finding might be that sleep apnea is common in obese women with PCOS [49]; androgen excess and subnormal estrogen levels and visceral adiposity may be involved in sleep disturbances [50].

4.2.3 Eating Disorders

Association between PCOS and eating disorder has been suggested, mainly correlated to the body image dissatisfaction. 6 % of women with PCOS fall into the bulimic range [51], and moreover, PCOS was more frequently found among bulimic women [52]. Compared to the general population, eating disorders seem to be more prevalent in PCOS population: 12.6 % bulimia and 1.6 % anorexia.

Moreover, an epidemiological cohort study of eating disorders among hirsute women showed a high prevalence of untreated eating disorders, especially EDNOS (eating disorders not otherwise specified) and bulimia nervosa; hirsute women with an eating disorder had high levels of comorbid depression and anxiety: they suffered from lower self-esteem and considered themselves as more hirsute than they really were [53].

References

1. Farrell K, Antoni MH (2010) Insulin resistance, obesity, inflammation, and depression in polycystic ovary syndrome: biobehavioral mechanism and interventions. Fertil Steril 94:1565–1574
2. Spitzer RL, Kroenke K, Williams JB (1999) Validation and utility of a self-report version of PRIME-MD: the PHQ primary care study. JAMA 282:1737–1744
3. Kerchner A, Lester W, Stuart S, Dokras A (2009) Risk of depression and other mental health disorders in women with polycystic ovary syndrome: a longitudinal study. Fert Steril 91:207–212
4. Barnard L, Ferriday D, Guenther N et al (2007) Quality of life and psychological well being in polycystic ovary syndrome. Hum Reprod 22:2279–2286
5. Coffey S, Bano G, Mason HD (2006) Health-related quality of life in women with polycystic ovary syndrome: a comparison with the general population using the Polycystic Ovary Syndrome Questionnaire (PCOSQ) and the Short-Form-36 (SF-36). Gynecol Endocrinol 22:80–86
6. McCook JG, Reame N, Thatcher S (2005) Health-related quality of life issues in women with polycystic ovary syndrome. JOGNN 34:12–20
7. Elsenbruch S, Hahn S, Kowalsky D et al (2004) Quality of life, psychological well-being, and sexual satisfaction in women with polycystic ovary syndrome. J Clin Endocrinol Metab 88:5801–5807
8. Bazarganipour F, Ziaei S, Ali M et al (2013) Predictive factors of health-related quality of life in patients with polycystic ovary syndrome: a structural equation modeling approach. Fertil Steril 100(5):1389–1396

9. De Niet JE, De Koning CM, Pastoor H et al (2010) Psychological well-being and sexarche in women with polycystic ovary syndrome. Hum Reprod 25:1497–1503

10. Brown PJ (1991) Culture and evolution of obesity. Hum Nat 2:57

11. Deurenberg P, Deurenberg-Yap M, Guricci S (2002) Asians are different from Caucasians and from each other in their body mass index/body fat per cent relationship. Obes Rev 3:141–146

12. Guyatt G, Weaver B, Cronin L et al (2004) Health-related quality of life in women with polycystic ovary syndrome, a self-administered questionnaire, was validated. J Clin Epidemiol 57:1279–1287

13. Kitzinger C, Willmott J (2002) The thief of womanhood: women's experience of polycystic ovary syndrome. Soc Sci Med 54:349–361

14. Willmott J (2000) The experiences of women with polycystic ovary syndrome. Fem Psychol 10:107–116

15. Farkas J, Rigò A, Zsolt D (2014) Psychological aspects of the polycystic ovary syndrome. Gynecol Endocrinol 30(2):95–99

16. Ekback M, Wijma K, Benzein E (2009) It is always on my mind: women's experience of their bodies when living with hirsutism. Health Care Women Int 30:358–372

17. Lipton MG, Sherr L, Elford J et al (2006) Women living with facial hair: the psychological and behavioral burden. J Psychosom Res 61:161–168

18. Elsenbruch S, Benson S, Hahn S (2006) Reply: incorporating qualitative approaches is the path to adequate understanding of the psychosocial impact of polycystic ovary syndrome. Hum Reprod 21:2724–2725

19. Trent M, Rich M, Bryn Austin A, Gordon C (2003) Fertility concerns and sexual behavior in adolescent girls with polycystic ovary syndrome: implications for quality of life. J Pediatr Adolesc Gynecol 16:33–37

20. Omran AR (1992) Family planning in the legacy of Islam. Routledge, London

21. Gottlieb A (1982) Sex, fertility and menstruation among the Beng of the Ivory Coast: a symbolic analysis. Africa (Lond) 52:3447–3466

22. Gorzynski G, Katz JL (1977) The polycystic ovary syndrome: psychosexual correlates. Arch Sex Behav 6:215–222

23. Mansson M, Norstrom K et al (2011) Sexuality and psychological wellbeing in women with polycystic ovary syndrome compared with healthy controls. Eur J Obst Gyn Reprod Biol 155:161–165

24. American Psychiatric Association. Diagnostic and statistical manual of mental disorders, 4th edn – Text Revision (DSM-IV-TR) (2000) Washington, DC

25. Dokras A, Clifton S, Futterweit W, Wild R (2012) Increased prevalence of anxiety symptoms in women with polycystic ovary syndrome: systematic review and meta-analysis. Fertil Steril 97:225–230

26. Weiner CL, Primeau M, Ehrmann DA (2004) Androgens and mood dysfunction in women: comparison of women with polycystic ovarian syndrome to healthy controls. Psychosom Med 66:356–362

27. Rasgon NL, Rao RC, Hwang S et al (2003) Depression in women with polycystic ovary syndrome: clinical and biochemical correlates. J Affect Disord 74:299–304

28. Keegan A, Liao L-M, Boyle M (2003) Hirsutism: a psychological analysis. J Health Psychol 8(3):327–345

29. Bernestein J, Potts N, Mattox JH (1985) Assessment of psychological dysfunction associated with infertility. J Obst Gynecol Neonatal Nurs 14(Suppl 6):S63–S66

30. Bernestein J, Brill M, Levin S, Seibel M (1992) Coping with infertility: a new nursing perspective. NAACOG's Clin Issues Perinatal Womens Health Nurs 3:335–342

31. Bodner C, Garratt A, Ratcliffe J et al (1997) Measuring health-related quality of life outcomes in women with endometriosis: results of the gynaecology audit project in Scotland. Health Bull (Edinburgh) 55:109–117

32. Mansson M, Holte J, Landin-Wilhemsen K et al (2008) Women with polycystic ovary syndrome are often depressed or anxious: a case control study. Psychoneuroendocrinology 33:1132–1138

33. Hollinrake E, Abreu A, Maifeld M et al (2007) Increased risk of depressive disorders in women with polycystic ovary syndrome. Fertil Steril 87(6):1369–1376
34. Azziz R, Woods KS, Rena R (2004) The prevalence and features of the polycystic ovary syndrome in an unselected population. J Clin Endocrinol Metab 89:2745–2749
35. Benson S, Hahn S, Tan S et al (2009) Prevalence and implications of anxiety in polycystic ovary syndrome: results of an internet-based survey in Germany. Hum Reprod 24:1446–1451
36. Roberts RE, Deleger S, Strawbridge WJ, Kaplan GA (2003) Prospective association between obesity and depression: evidence from the Alameda County study. Int J Obes 27:514–521
37. Ramasubbu R (2002) Insulin resistance: a metabolic link between depressive disorder and atherosclerotic vascular disease. Med Hypothesis 59:537–551
38. Brown AJ (2004) Depression and insulin resistance: applications to polycystic ovary syndrome. Clin Obstet Gynecol 47:592–596
39. Dokras A (2012) Mood and anxiety disorders in women with PCOS. Steroids 77:338–341
40. Jedel E, Waem M, Gustafson D et al (2010) Anxiety and depression symptoms in women with polycystic ovary syndrome compared with controls matched for body mass index. Hum Reprod 25:450–456
41. Yazici K, Baz K, Yazici AE et al (2004) Disease-specific quality of life is associated with anxiety and depression in patients with acne. J Eur Acad Dermatol 18:435–439
42. Petry NM, Barry D, Pietrzak RH, Wagner JA (2008) Overweight and obesity are associated with psychiatric disorders: results from the National Epidemiologic Survey on Alcohol and Related Conditions. Psychosom Med 70:288–297
43. Lechner L, Bolman C, van Dalen A (2007) Definite involuntary childlessness: associations between coping, social support and psychological distress. Hum Reprod 22:288–294
44. Britten N (1995) Qualitative interviews in medical research. Br Med J 311:251–253
45. Livadas S, Chaskou S, Kandaraki AA et al (2011) Anxiety is associated with hormonal and metabolic profile in women with polycystic ovarian syndrome. Clin Endocrinol (Oxf) 75:698–703
46. Drosdzol A, Skrzypulec V, Plinta R (2010) Quality of life, mental health and self-esteem in hirsute adolescent females. J Psychosom Obstet Gynaecol 31:168–175
47. Clayton WJ, Lipton M, Elford J et al (2005) A randomized controlled trial of laser treatment among hirsute women with polycystic ovary syndrome. Br J Dermatol 152:986–992
48. Jones GL, Balen AH, Ledger WL (2008) Health-related quality of life in PCOS and related infertility: how can we assess this? Hum Fertil 11(3):173–185
49. Vgontzas AN, Legro RS, Bixler EO et al (2001) Polycystic ovary syndrome is associated with obstructive sleep apnea and daytime sleepiness: role of insulin resistance. J Clin Endocrinol Metab 86:517–520
50. Tasali E, Van Cauter E, Ehrmann DA (2008) Polycystic ovary syndrome and obstructive sleep apnea. Sleep Med Clin 3:37–46
51. Jahanfar S, Eden JA, Nguyen TV (1995) Bulimia nervosa and the polycystic ovary syndrome. Gynecol Endocrinol 9:113–117
52. Raphael FJ, Rodin DA, Peattie A (1995) Ovarian morphology and insulin sensitivity in women with bulimia nervosa. Clin Endocrinol 43:451–455
53. Morgan J, Scholtz S, Lacey H, Conway G (2008) The prevalence of eating disorders in women with facial hirsutism: an epidemiological cohort study. Int J Eat Disord 41:427–431

Diagnosis and Assessment

5

Currently the ESHRE/ASRM or Rotterdam criteria are the agreed international diagnostic criteria for PCOS [1].

PCOS diagnosis can be raised only after the exclusion of other known causes of hyperandrogenism and amenorrhea and when there are at least two of the three following parameters:

1. Oligomenorrhea or anovulatory cycles with menstrual irregularities
2. Elevated levels of circulating androgens or clinical manifestation of hyperandrogenism
3. Ultrasound evidence of micropolycystic ovaries

5.1 Differential Diagnosis

First of all, to establish a differential diagnosis is a primary goal when a patient complains of menstrual disorders, infertility, hyperandrogenism, and overweight/obesity, in order to identify all possible clinical scenarios that are characterized by symptoms and signs similar to PCOS features.

These are the following:

- Hyperprolactinemia: history of galactorrhea, spontaneous or induced.
- Thyroid dysfunctions: frequent symptoms are hot or cold intolerance, tremors, diffuse scalp hair loss, weight change, and textural skin changes.
- Ovarian/adrenal androgen-secreting tumors: symptoms of deep virilization such as increased libido, deepened voice, and clitoromegaly.
- Non-classic congenital adrenal 21-hydroxylase deficiency: this disorder is caused by a partial adrenal enzyme defect that leads to impaired cortisol production, compensatory elevation in adrenocorticotropic hormone, and subsequent excess androgen production. Premature pubarche could be a clue symptom.

© Springer International Publishing Switzerland 2015
M. Stracquadanio, L. Ciotta, *Metabolic Aspects of PCOS: Treatment with Insulin Sensitizers*, DOI 10.1007/978-3-319-16760-2_5

- Cushing's syndrome: late-onset hirsutism, mood or sleep disturbance, hyperpigmented striae, easy bruising, thin/fragile skin, facial plethora, supraclavicular fullness, excessive thirst, and increased susceptibility to infections.
- Virilizing drugs: anabolic steroids, glucocorticoids, valproic acid, etc.
- Simple obesity.
- Premature ovarian failure or stress amenorrhea.

It is important to assess the onset and evolution of hyperandrogenism signs because a rapid onset (2–6 months) is suspicious of androgen-secreting neoplasms, while a slow onset and evolution (especially during the adolescence) is more peculiar of PCOS. Moreover, it is relevant to investigate the possible intake of virilizing drugs.

## 5.2	Risk Factors

Anamnesis is important to assess the presence of various risk factors, such as:

- Family medical history positive for:
  - Type II diabetes
  - Hyperandrogenism
  - Impaired glucose tolerance
  - Hyperinsulinemia
  - Obesity
  - Metabolic syndrome
  - Preeclampsia
  - Gestational diabetes
- Personal medical history positive for:
  - Early pubarche
  - Overweight/obesity
  - Macrosomia
  - Sedentary lifestyle
  - Poor dietary habits

## 5.3	Clinical–Endocrine Features

### 5.3.1	Oligomenorrhea and Anovulation

Oligomenorrhea is defined as menstrual periods occurring at intervals of greater than 35 days, with only four to nine periods in a year.

During the early post-menarche years, the menstrual cycles can last between 21 and 45 days [2]. The characteristic menstrual regularity of the adult female is usually reached several years following menarche; according to some studies, the persistent presence of cycles longer than 45 days, 3–5 years following the menarche, suggests the presence of ovulatory dysfunction in adolescent girls [3].

Progesterone levels <5 ng/mL in days 20–24 (luteal phase) of the menstrual cycle is a good cutoff to diagnose an anovulatory cycle. In contrast, a patient can be diagnosed as anovulatory after ascertaining anovulation in at least two subsequent cycles, in the presence of hypoprogesteronemia.

5.3.2 Hirsutism

Hirsutism can be assessed through the Ferriman–Gallwey score [4] that evaluates the presence of the terminal hair in the upper lip, chin, chest, upper and lower back, upper and lower abdomen, thighs, and arms.

A score of 0–4 is assigned to each area examined, based on the visual density of terminal hairs, such that a score of 0 represents the absence of terminal hairs, a score of 1 minimally evident terminal hair growth, and a score of 4 extensive terminal hair growth. Terminal hairs can be distinguished clinically from vellus hairs primarily by their length (i.e., >0.5 cm), coarseness, and pigmentation. On the contrary, vellus hairs generally measure <0.5 cm in length and are soft and nonpigmented.

Integrated scores from all body areas beyond 15 points are related to a hirsutism diagnosis, although current recommendations suggest the use of 95th percentile of the score in specific populations, adapting to ethnic groups, hair pattern, and age-related features, in order to properly diagnose hirsutism [4].

This score system has limitations because of the subjective nature of the assessments and the difficulty of evaluating women who have cosmetically removed their hairs [5].

Moreover, the F–G score was developed in Caucasian adult women and may not be applicable to younger women from different ethnic backgrounds (e.g., for Indian women) [6].

5.3.3 Acne

The two commonly used measures to assess the severity of acne are grading and lesion counting, but no grading system has been universally accepted [7].

In 1956, Pillsbury, Shelley, and Kligman published the earliest known grading system [8], which includes the following:

- Grade 1: comedones and occasional small cysts confined to the face
- Grade 2: comedones with occasional pustules and small cysts confined to the face
- Grade 3: many comedones and small and large inflammatory papules and pustules, more extensive but confined to the face
- Grade 4: many comedones and deep lesions tending to coalescence and canalize and involving the face and the upper aspects of the trunk

A more recent and complete system is the one created, in 1997, by Doshi, Zaheer, and Stiller [9], called "Global Acne Grading System (GAGS)". This system divides the face, chest, and back into six areas (forehead, each cheek, nose, chin, chest, and back) and assigns a factor to each area on the basis of size.

Each type of lesion is given a value depending on severity:

- No lesions = 0
- Comedones = 1
- Papules = 2
- Pustules = 3
- Nodules = 4

The score for each area (local score) is calculated using the formula:

$$\text{Local Score} = \text{Factor} \times \text{Grade}\ (0-4)$$

The global score is the sum of local scores, and acne severity was graded using the global score. A score of 1–18 is considered mild; 19–30, moderate; 31–38, severe; and >39, very severe.

5.4   Endocrine Blood Tests

Blood tests should be done within 10 days from the beginning of a menstrual cycle, during the early follicular phase. Many studies suggest that hyperandrogenemia may be the most useful diagnostic feature in adolescents because menstrual irregularities, ovarian morphology, and clinical hyperandrogenism do not correlate strongly with PCOS in this population [10, 11], even if there is a physiological increase in androgen levels during puberty [12, 13].

The following are the blood substrates and their values characteristic of PCOS.

As explained previously, in the meanwhile, it is crucial to assess other blood values (TSH, fT3, fT4, anti-TPO, anti-Tg, prolactin, DHEAS, 24 h urinary cortisol and creatinine) in order to exclude other pathologies:

- LH $\geq$10 mUI/mL
- LH/FSH ratio $\geq$2.5
- Estradiol $\geq$30 pg/mL
- 17-OHP $\leq$2 ng/mL
  If the value is >2 ng/mL (6 nmol/l), it is suspicious of non-classic congenital adrenal 21-hydroxylase deficiency (NCAH), and ACTH test is required: it is an acute adrenal stimulation test that measures 17-OHP before and 60 min after the intravenous administration of an adrenocorticotropic hormone analog. If the

stimulated 17-OHP exceeds 30 nmol/l, and preferably 45 nmol/l, the diagnosis of NCAH is confirmed [14].

- Androstenedione $\geq$2.5 ng/mL
- SHBG $\leq$15 nmol/l
- Testosterone $\geq$1 ng/mL

 A serum testosterone level >200 ng/dL is highly suggestive of an adrenal or ovarian tumor. If serum testosterone is elevated despite a normal DHEAS level, an ovarian source is more likely. If a DHEAS level >700 mcg/dL is present despite a normal serum testosterone level, an adrenal source should be suspected as the cause of hirsutism [4].

 Mildly elevated serum testosterone and DHEAS are often present in functional ovarian hyperandrogenism (FOH) and late-onset congenital adrenal hyperplasia (CAH).

 A very recent study has revealed that PCOS patients with co-elevation of androstenedione and testosterone have impaired indices of insulin sensitivity compared with those with normal androgens or milder hyperandrogenemia [15].

- *FAI*: free androgen index or FAI is a ratio used to determine abnormal androgen status in humans. The ratio is the total testosterone level divided by the sex hormone-binding globulin (SHBG) level and then multiplying by a constant, usually 100. The concentrations of testosterone and SHBG are normally measured in nanomoles per liter, while FAI has no units [16, 17].

$$FAI = 100 \times \left(Total\ Testosterone / SHBG \right)$$

The majority of testosterone in the blood does not exist as free molecule, while half is tightly bound to sex hormone-binding globulin, and the other half is weakly bound to albumin. Only a small percentage is unbound (<3 % in females and <0.7 % in males). Since only free testosterone is able to bind to tissue receptors to exercise its effects, it is believed that free testosterone is the best marker of a person's androgen status. However, free testosterone is difficult and expensive to measure, and many laboratories do not offer this service.

The free androgen index is intended to give a guide to the free testosterone level, but it is not very accurate. Consequently, there are no universally agreed "normal ranges," and levels slightly above or below quoted laboratory reference ranges may not be clinically significant.

Typical values for the FAI in women are 7–10 [18].

- A serum *AMH $\geq$35 pmol/l (or $\geq$5 ng/mL)* appears to be more sensitive and specific than a USS follicle count >19 [19].

 There is not yet an international consortium that validates the threshold for AMH. In another recent study, Lin et al. have divided all patients into three groups: high AMH (>11 ng/mL), moderate AMH (4–11 ng/mL), and low AMH (<4 ng/mL). As the AMH level increased, the prevalence of PCOS increased significantly from 21 % in the low-AMH group to 37 % in the moderate-AMH group and 80 % in the high-AMH group [20].

5.5 Ultrasound Features

Polycystic ovarian morphology (PCOM) is an important element for the diagnosis of polycystic ovarian syndrome in adult women. The Rotterdam consensus defined PCOM as the presence of 12 or more follicles of 2–9 mm in diameter and/or an ovarian volume greater than 10 mL in at least 1 ovary (Fig. 5.1).

Some studies have shown that a combination of these characteristics is better than one, to give greater sensitivity and specificity [21–23].

The subjective aspect of the ovaries, their follicular distribution, or the appearance of the stroma is not considered as important:

- *Ovarian volume*: there are many formulas available for the calculation of ovarian volume, but investigators stated that it should be calculated on the basis of the simplified formula for an ellipsoid: 0.5 × length × width × thickness of the ovary [21, 23–25].
- *Number of follicles*: the adoption of the above-cited criterion for defining a polycystic ovary is different from the methodology used in prior works, which attempted to define PCOM on the basis of the presence of at least ten follicles arranged peripherally around an echodense stroma [26] in a single US imaging plane. The key technical requirement for the assessment of the number of follicles is that the number of antral follicles present throughout the entire volume of the ovary must be counted [27].
- *Stromal echogenicity and volume*: one of the features of polycystic ovary is the increased stromal echogenicity [26]. However, the intrinsic echogenicity of the ovarian stroma is no different in PCOS than in the normal ovary; the subjective impression of increased stromal echogenicity is due to the increased stromal

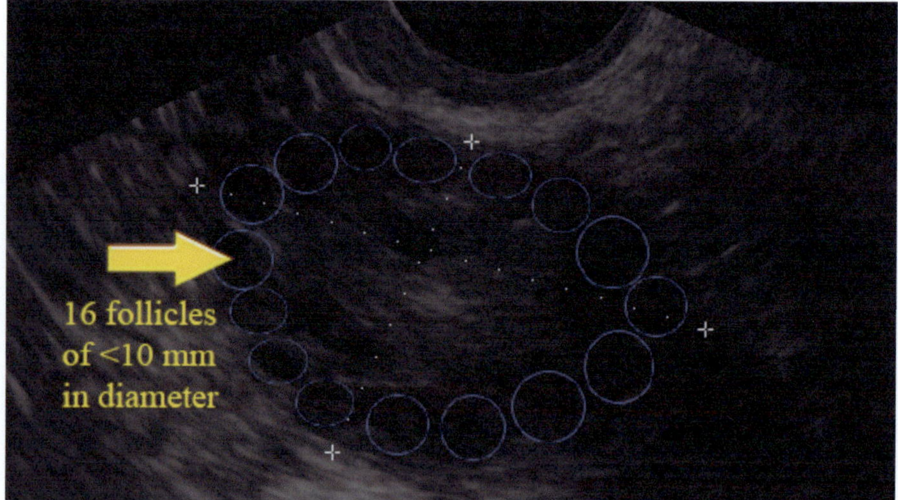

Fig. 5.1 Polycystic ovarian morphology

volume, which positively correlates with serum androgen levels [28]. At the moment, no standardized method is available for this determination. Because overall ovarian volume correlates well with stromal volume in polycystic ovaries [28] and is more easily to evaluate, the determination of overall ovarian volume is a reliable surrogate for ovarian stromal assessment [27].

Moreover, the Rotterdam consensus states that, wherever possible, ultrasounds should be carried out endo-vaginally particularly in obese patients [1] because of its better resolution in comparison to the transabdominal route.

In fact, data suggest that, compared with transvaginal US, the appearance of polycystic ovaries may not be detected at transabdominal US in up to 30 % of women with PCOS [29].

All ultrasounds have to be carried out in the early follicular phase (3rd–6th day) in women with regular menstrual cycles or in patients with oligomenorrhea (often after MAP test); in case of amenorrhea, the study can be carried out on any given day.

A history of oral contraceptive use should be obtained, since oral contraceptive use causes a decrease in ovarian size, decreasing the sensitivity of US evaluation.

The above-reported criteria are of limited value in the adolescent population [30]. In primis, transvaginal USS is inappropriate in virginal patients, diminishing the quality of imaging obtained [31]. Moreover, ovarian morphology changes during the lifespan, with a maximum size and antral follicle count around menarche [32, 33]: in fact, the mean ovarian volume is larger in young women. The consensus group also cites the difficulty in distinguishing a polycystic ovary from what has traditionally been referred to as a multifollicular ovary, defined as an ovary in which there are six or more follicles (usually 4–10 mm in diameter) with normal stromal echogenicity and described as the common appearance of ovaries in adolescents [26]. Given these physiological features, many adolescents might meet the adult criteria for PCOM [34]. For the explained reasons, there is a lack of high quality evidence on which to base a recommendation on appropriate criteria for ultrasound diagnosis of PCOM in adolescents [30]: thus, USS results should be interpreted with caution [34].

Moreover, it is known that ovarian volume and follicle number decrease linearly with age in women with PCOS and controls, but some studies showed that the follicle number was higher at all ages in PCOS compared with control women [35, 36]: thus, regarding the follicle number count, it is necessary to create an age-based criteria to define PCOM [33].

On the other hand, some studies showed that these ultrasonographic findings are frequent in young women and decrease with age [33, 37, 38]. In adults, these USS findings may be present in 10–20 % of healthy women with regular menstrual cycles and without clinical hyperandrogenism [39, 40].

Other data suggest that 23 % of women of reproductive age will have findings of PCOM [39] and only 5–10 % of these patients will have classic symptoms of PCOS [41].

The use of polycystic ovaries as an inclusion/exclusion criterion for a diagnostic test study is controversial; much of the debates, in fact, have arisen from reports of unusually high rates of polycystic ovaries in healthy women of reproductive age using the ultrasound-based criteria supported by the Rotterdam consensus [38].

According to a very recent study, an average value of 26 or more follicles per ovary is a reliable threshold for detecting PCOM in women with frank symptoms of PCOS; a lower follicle threshold may be required to detect milder variants of the syndrome [42].

Thus, given the significant number of women of reproductive age who have PCOM as defined on the basis of US criteria, actually it would be ideal and prudent to write this observation in the report: "Findings meet the Rotterdam Consensus definition for polycystic ovaries. In the absence of ovulatory dysfunction or either clinically or biochemically diagnosed hyperandrogenism, findings are not specific and do not indicate the presence of polycystic ovarian syndrome" [27].

Summarizing, Lee and Rausch in a recent study propose the "pertinent USS reporting parameters in PCOS" [27]:

- Separate reporting for each ovary
- Number and size range of follicles
- Size of the largest follicle should be measured in three axes and the average diameter calculated
- Documentation of any follicle >10 mm or corpus luteum (presence of either suggest the necessity of repeating USS during the next menstrual cycle)
- Ovarian volume, calculated with the simplified formula for an ellipsoid: (0.5 × length × width × thickness)

5.6 Clinical–Metabolic Features

As largely explained in the previous chapters, a metabolic evaluation is necessary for every PCOS patient. From a clinical–metabolic point of view, physician should:

1. Observe the presence of obesity and evaluate the distribution of body fat (gynoid or android) by assessing
   - *BMI* = weight / height^2 kg/m^2 (Table 5.1)
   - *Waist/hip ratio (WHR)* >0.80
     According to the World Health Organization [43], the waist circumference (WC) should be measured at the midpoint between the lower margin of the last palpable rib and the top of the iliac crest, using a stretch-resistant tape that provides a constant 100 g tension. WC should be <88 cm.
     Hip circumference should be measured around the widest portion of the buttocks, with the tape parallel to the floor [44].
     WHR and BMI are the easiest anthropometric indices to use in clinical practice to check the effects of adipose tissue on the metabolic profile. However, BMI and WHR are indirect methods of assessing body composition and, in some cases, inaccurate, but they permit a first diagnostic level.

Table 5.1 WHO—weight and BMI classification

Weight classification	BMI (kg/m^2) cutoff
Underweight	<18.5
Mild thinness	<16
Moderate thinness	16–16.9
Severe thinness	17–18.4
Normal range	18.5–24.9
Overweight	≥25
Pre-obese	25–29.9
Obesity	≥30
Obese—class I	30–34.9
Obese—class II	35–39.9
Obese—class III	≥40

Particularly, waist circumference should be examined in every PCOS patient with normal BMI, to identify individuals at higher risk for developing metabolic disorders [45].

- Recently, a Brazilian study group tried to develop equations that utilize *anthropometric measures* to estimate intra-abdominal fat (IAF) and total abdominal fat (TAF) in obese women with PCOS [46]. The anthropometric variables used are AC (abdominal circumference), WC (waist circumference), CC (chest circumference), and NC (neck circumference):
  - Abdominal circumference (AC): it was measured at the point corresponding to the navel.
  - Waist circumference (WC): the patient was asked to stand upright, and a measure of the smallest curvature between the ribs and the iliac crest was taken without compressing the tissues [47].
  - Trunk circumference (TC): it is measured on the posterior part of the trunk, 3 cm under the armpit. The patient must place her arms parallel to the body [48].
  - Neck circumference (NC): it must be measured at the upper margin of the thyroid cartilage [49].

  The model proposed for TAF was: $4.63725 + 0.01483 \times AC - 0.00117 \times NC - 0.00177 \times CC$ ($R^2 = 0.78$); the model proposed for IAF was: $1.88541 + 0.01878 \times WC + 0.05687 \times NC - 0.01529 \times CC$ ($R^2 = 0.51$).

  Authors showed that these equations had good correlation with the real value measured by CT scan and so can be used in clinical practice [46].

- A Korean study group proposed the *visceral adiposity index (VAI)* to reflect visceral adiposity and insulin resistance. It is a mathematical model that uses simple anthropometric (BMI and WC) and functional (triglycerides and HDL) parameters [50].

  The VAI is calculated using the following formula: $\left[WC / \left(36.58 + \left(1.89 \times BMI \right) \right) \right] \times \left(TG / 0.81 \right) \times \left(1.52 / HDL \right)$, where the triglycerides and HDL concentrations are expressed in mmol/l [50].

  This study observed that the VAI was an independent determinant of visceral adiposity and can replace visceral CT scanning [51].

More than these indirect methods, there are also different direct imaging techniques, more sophisticated and accurate, such as DEXA, MRI, CT scan, impedentiometry, and ultrasound scan.

- *DEXA (dual-energy X-ray absorptiometry)*: it is based on the ability of the tissues to attenuate a dual-energy-level photon beam (70 and 140 kV), according to the mass and density of the tissue passed through. Currently DEXA is considered a reliable test for the assessment of body composition (BF%) because of its high sensitivity and reproducibility in the quantification of lean and fat mass, both in the whole body and region by region; thus, DEXA is extremely useful for the assessment of body fat distribution and allows an accurate distinction between abdominal fat (android) and gluteal–femoral fat (gynoid).

  Moreover, it is a method without any radiological risk, as the photon beam is collimated and the exposure dose emitted is minimal (<1 mrem). Accordingly, it is an investigation that can be frequently repeated, in order to do a very close control of the body.

  On the other hand, a recent study reported that BMI and WC were more accurate than BF% for classifying the studied metabolic disorders. The BF% cutoffs most frequently cited by international scientific literature are BF% $\geq$30 and BF% $\geq$35 for women: they produce a high rate of false positives [52].

- *CT scan*: CT scan, compared to DEXA, offers the advantage of a discrimination between subcutaneous and visceral fat, and it is able to quantify the proportion of fatty tissue that best correlates with cardiovascular and metabolic risk, which is the visceral fat.

  The adipose tissue areas are calculated by computing the fat area surfaces with an attenuation range of −190 to −30 Hounsfield units. The abdominal visceral fat area (VFA) is measured by drawing a line in the muscle wall surrounding the abdominal cavity, at the level of L4–L5 vertebral bodies [53].

  The cutoff value of visceral fat area associated with an increase risk of obesity-related disorder, according to the literature, is 103.8 cm [2] (sensitivity 74.5 %, specificity 64.7 %) [54].

  Thus, women with VFA >100 cm^2 are at high risk of metabolic syndrome [51].

  However, the high cost, long scan times (possible artifacts due to involuntary movements by the patient), and exposure to a non-negligible radiological risk constitute a strong limitation, and so a repeated use for the measurement of body composition is not recommended.

- *Impedentiometry*: this method estimates the body composition based on the physical principle of the different electrical conduction of the tissues, in relation to their content of water and electrolytes. The conduction of an electric current is in fact much higher in lean than fat tissue. By applying a weak electrical current to the body and detecting the impedance presented by the body itself to the passage of this current, it is possible to calculate the quantity of total body water (TBW). The advantages of this technique are easy way to use, the absolute noninvasiveness, and measurement speed. The limitations of the method relate to the situations with changes in hydration body and/or in the electrolyte concentration.

2. Finally, from a clinical–metabolic point of view, the physician should verify the presence of hypertension or clinical signs of hyperinsulinemia such as *acanthosis nigricans (AN)*.

   AN is a skin lesion appearing thickened and velvety brown streaking to a leathery, verrucous, papillomatous change. It usually occurs on the neck or in skinfolds. Microscopically, AN is characterized by an increased number of melanocytes, with papillary hypertrophy and hyperkeratosis [45]. Benign acanthosis nigricans usually correlates to insulin resistance or obesity [55, 56].

   A very recent Chinese study showed that the presence of AN correlates to insulin resistance and reduced HDL-C level in PCOS patients with normal BMI. Because of its easy identification, AN could be a reliable marker of IR, but it lacks the sensitivity to become a noninvasive diagnostic tool for IR in women with normal BMI [45].

5.7 Metabolic Blood Tests

As reported previously, ~50–70 % of women with PCOS are characterized by hyperinsulinemic insulin resistance, which plays a causative role in the development of the metabolic syndrome.

The American College of Obstetricians and Gynecologists currently recommends screening women with PCOS for glucose intolerance and lipid abnormalities.

> **Metabolic Blood Tests Recommended in PCOS Women**
> - OGTT (biannual rescreening) or HOMA-IR
> - Total cholesterol + LDL-C + HDL-C
> - Triglycerides
> - Transaminases

5.7.1 Glucose Metabolism Assessment and Calculation of Insulin Resistance

First of all, a correct evaluation of carbohydrate metabolism is necessary, and so it is important to remember which are the normal glycemic and insulinemic values.

- Fasting glycemia:
  - Normal, 70–100 mg/dL
  - "Grey zone," 100–126 mg/dL
  - Diabetes, >126 mg/dL
- Fasting insulinemia: <10 mUI/mL

The World Health Organization (WHO) criteria for impaired fasting glucose (IFG) differ from the American Diabetes Association (ADA) criteria because the normal range of glucose is differently defined.

The WHO has defined the upper limit of normal at less than 110 mg/dL.

However, fasting glucose levels of 100 mg/dL and higher have been shown to significantly increase complication rates, and so the ADA has accordingly lowered the upper normal limit to a fasting glucose under 100 mg/dL.

- WHO IFG criteria: fasting plasma glucose level from 6.1 mmol/l (110 mg/dL) to 7 mmol/l (126 mg/dL).
- ADA IFG criteria: fasting plasma glucose level from 5.6 mmol/l (100 mg/dL) to 7 mmol/l (126 mg/dL) [57].
- *OGTT (oral glucose tolerance test)*: the most accurate method to diagnose insulin resistance is the OGTT after 75 g glucose challenge, even in adolescent women [58]. Normal values are the following:
  - Glycemia:
    - Fasting, 70–100 mg/dL
    - 60 min after glucose administration, <180 mg/dL
    - 120 min after glucose administration, <140 mg/dL

Impaired glucose tolerance (IGT) is defined when glucose level is >140 mg/dL 2 h after glucose load, but <200 mg/dL.

Diabetes is defined when glycemia is >200 mg/dL 2 h after glucose load.

  - Insulinemia:
    - Fasting, <10 mUI/mL
    - 60 min after glucose administration, <60 mUI/mL
    - 120 min after glucose administration, ≈10 mUI/mL

Of course, the majority of PCOS patients are not diabetic yet, but only insulin resistant; insulin resistance is defined when insulin value 1 h after OGTT is >60 mUI/mL and/or its level is not very close to the fasting insulin value after 2 h post-glucose administration.

It has been suggested that an OGTT should be performed every 2 years for those with normal glucose tolerance and annually if IFG or IGT is present [59].

Glucose screening recommendations for PCOS women are summarized in Table 5.2

- *HOMA index*: OGTT is not a very confortable method, and it is also expensive and time-consuming; for this reason, the need for a simple way of measuring insulin resistance has led to the creation of a large number of insulin sensitivity indices [60, 61]. The most used model is the HOMA index.

The homeostatic model for assessment of insulin resistance (HOMA-IR) is a simple and noninvasive method of estimating insulin sensitivity from the steady glucose and insulin concentrations measured under fasting conditions.

It was calculated using the following formula [62]:

$$\text{Fasting glycemia}\left(\text{mmol}/l\right) \times \text{Fasting insulinemia}\left(\text{mUI}/\text{mL}\right)/22.5$$

Table 5.2 Glucose assessment in PCOS patients—screening recommendations

AACE (American Association of Clinical Endocrinologists) ACE (American College of Endocrinology)	OGTT for all PCOS patients aged >30 year. Periodically reassess
RCOG (Royal College of Obstetricians and Gynaecologists)	Screen all by fasting glucose regularly. If fasting glucose >100 mg/dL or BMI >30 kg/m^2 or positive family history, screen by OGTT
ACOG (American College of Obstetricians and Gynecologists)	OGTT for all women with PCOS. Repeat every 2 years
AE-PCOS (Androgen Excess and Polycystic Ovary Syndrome Society)	OGTT for PCOS women with BMI >30 kg/m^2 or in lean women with advanced age (>40 years), personal history of gestational diabetes, or family history of diabetes mellitus type II

HOMA index values for percentiles 50–75 ranged from 2.07 to 2.83 [63].

- *Glucose/insulin ratio*: this simple measure of insulin resistance in PCOS women has been correlated well with more complicated dynamic tests of insulin action [64].
  It has been reported that a fasting G:I ratio of 4.5 or less is a measure of IR in obese PCOS women, and this cutoff value has a sensitivity of 95 %, specificity of 84 %, positive predictive value of 87 %, and negative predictive value of 94 % [65].
- *Diabetes screening*
  Recently, a study group from Holland proposed a stepwise screening for glucose metabolism abnormalities by fasting glucose for all women with PCOS and subsequent OGTT screening for diabetes in the small proportion of PCOS women with fasting glucose concentration between 110 and 126 mg/dL only, without compromising early diagnosis of diabetes [66].
  However, validation of this new screening algorithm is waited.
  Previously, it has been shown that fasting glucose rather than OGTT underestimates the prevalence of diabetes mellitus type II in PCOS women by >50 % [67].
  Hemoglobin A1c is a commonly used marker of chronic glycemia, and it reflects the average blood glucose levels over a 2–3-month period [68].
  ADA suggests HbA1c levels as a screening tool for diabetes and prediabetes in the general population with cutoff levels of 6.5 and 5.6 %, respectively [69], even if other studies stated that it is insensitive for prediabetes [68].

5.7.2   Lipid and Hepatic Profile

Dyslipidemia is common in PCOS and is present in up to 70 % of subjects [59, 70].

The AE-PCOS Society consensus statement [59] recommends a complete lipid and hepatic profile in all patients with PCOS. Pathological values are:

- Total cholesterol >200 mg/dL
- LDL cholesterol >130 mg/dL

- HDL cholesterol <50 mg/dL
- Triglycerides >150 mg/dL
- AST >30 U/l
- ALT >35 U/l
- γ-GT >38 U/l

The fatty liver index (FLI) is an algorithm based on BMI, waist circumference, triglycerides, and γ-GT and might serve as a simple and accurate predictor of hepatic steatosis in general population. FLI <30 rules out fatty liver disease, while FLI >60 indicates fatty liver disease [71]. FLI is calculated by the following formula:

$$\left(\frac{e^{0.953 \times \log e(\text{triglycerides}) + 0.139 \times \text{BMI} + 0.718 \times \log e(g-\text{GT}) + 0.053 \times \text{waist circumference} - 15.745}}{1 + e^{0.953 \times \log e(\text{triglycerides}) + 0.139 \times \text{BMI} + 0.718 \times \log e(g-\text{GT}) + 0.053 \times \text{waist circumference} - 15.745}} \right) \times 100$$

A recent study revealed that high FLI levels are a common finding in obese PCOS women and are closely linked to metabolic syndrome. Thus, FLI might be a useful index to identify PCOS women at high metabolic and hepatic risk in whom a very careful surveillance is needed and who might benefit from lifestyle counseling [72].

References

1. Rotterdam ESHRE/ASRM-Sponsored PCOS Consensus Workshop Group (2004) Revised (2003) consensus on diagnostic criteria and long- term health risks related to polycystic ovary syndrome. Fertil Steril 81:19–25
2. Diaz A, Laufer MR, Breech LL (2006) Menstruation in girls and adolescents: using the menstrual cycle as a vital sign. Pediatrics 118(5):2245–2250
3. Adams Hillard PJ (2008) Menstruation in adolescents: what's normal, what's not. Ann N Y Acad Sci 1135:29–35
4. Brodell LA, Mercurio MG (2010) Hirsutism: diagnosis and management. Gend Med 7(2):79–87
5. Blume-Peytavi U (2013) How to diagnose and treat medically women with excessive hair. Dermatol Clin 31:57–65
6. Biro FM, Emans SJ (2008) Whither PCOS? The challenges of establishing hyperandrogenism in adolescent girls. J Adolesc Health 43:103–105
7. Adityan B, Kumari R, Thappa DM (2009) Scoring systems in acne vulgaris. Indian J Dermatol Venereol Leprology 75:323–326
8. Witkowsky JA, Parish LC (2004) The assessment of acne: an evaluation of grading and lesion counting in the measurement of acne. Clin Dermatol 22:394–397
9. Doshi A, Zaheer A, Stiller MJ (1997) A comparison of current acne grading systems and proposal of a novel system. Int J Dermatol 36:416–418
10. Carmina E, Oberfield SE, Lobo RA (2010) The diagnosis of polycystic ovary syndrome in adolescents. Am J Obstet Gynecol 203:201.e1–201.e5
11. Roe AH, Dokras A (2011) The diagnosis of polycystic ovary syndrome in adolescents. Rev Obstet Gynecol 4(2):45–51
12. Rosner W, Auchus RJ, Azziz R et al (2007) Position statement: utility, limitations, and pitfalls in measuring testosterone: and Endocrine Society position statement. J Clin Endocrinol Metab 92(2):405–413

13. Rieder J, Santoro N, Cohen HW et al (2008) Body shape and size and insulin resistance as early clinical predictors of hyperandrogenic anovulation in ethnic minority adolescent girls. J Adolesc Health 43(2):115–124
14. Goodarzi MO, Dumesic DA, Chazenbalk G, Azziz R (2011) Polycystic ovary syndrome: etiology, pathogenesis and diagnosis. Nat Rev Endocrinol 7:219–231
15. O'Reilly MW et al (2014) Hyperandrogenemia predicts metabolic phenotype in polycystic ovary syndrome: the utility of serum androstenedione. J Clin Endocrinol Metab 99(3):1027–1036
16. Souter I, Sanchez LA, Perez M et al (2004) The prevalence of androgen excess among patients with minimal unwanted hair growth. Am J Obstet Gynecol 191:759–767
17. Mathur RS, Moody LO, Landgrebbe S, Williamson HO (1981) Plasma androgens and sex hormone binding globulin in the evaluation of hirsute patients. Fertil Steril 35:29–37
18. Ly LP, Handelsman DJ (2005) Empirical estimation of free testosterone from testosterone and sex hormone-binding globulin immunoassays. Eur J Endocrinol 152:471–478
19. Dewailly D, Gronier H et al (2011) Diagnosis of polycystic ovary syndrome (PCOS): revisiting the threshold values of follicle count on ultrasound and of the serum AMH level for the definition of polycystic ovaries. Hum Reprod 26(11):3123–3129
20. Lin YH, Chiu WC, Wu CH et al (2011) Anti-Mullerian hormone and polycystic ovary syndrome. Fertil Steril 96:230–235
21. Pache TD, Wladimiroff JW, Hop WCJ, Fauser BCJM (1992) How to discriminate between normal and polycystic ovaries: transvaginal US study. Radiology 183:421–423
22. Jonard S, Robert Y, Cortet-Rudelli C et al (2003) Ultrasound examination of polycystic ovaries: is it worth counting the follicles? Hum Reprod 18:598–603
23. Fulghesu AM, Ciampelli M, Belosi C et al (2001) A new ultrasound criterion for the diagnosis of polycystic ovary syndrome: the ovarian stroma/total area ratio. Fertil Steril 76:326–331
24. Swanson M, Sauerbrei EE, Cooperberg PL (1981) Medical implications of ultrasonically detected polycystic ovaries. J Clin Ultrasound 9(5):219–222
25. Saxton DW, Farquhar CM, Rae T, Beard RW (1990) Accuracy of ultrasound measurements of female pelvic organs. Br J Obstet Gynaecol 97(8):695–699
26. Adams J, Franks S, Polson DW et al (1985) Multifollicular ovaries: clinical and endocrine features and response to pulsatile gonadotropin releasing hormone. Lancet 2(8469–70):1375–1379
27. Lee TT, Rausch ME (2012) Polycystic ovarian syndrome: role of imaging in diagnosis. Radiographics 32:1643–1657
28. Kyei-Mensah AA, LinTan S, Zaidi J, Jacobs HS (1998) Relationship of ovarian stromal volume to serum androgen concentrations in patients with polycystic ovary syndrome. Hum Reprod 13(6):1437–1441
29. Fox R, Corrigan E, Thomas PA, Hull MG (1991) The diagnosis of polycystic ovaries in women with oligoamenorrhoea: predictive power of endocrine tests. Clin Endocrinol 34(2):127–131
30. Hardy TSE, Norman RJ (2013) Diagnosis of adolescent polycystic ovary syndrome. Steroids 78:751–754
31. Khan U (2007) Polycystic ovary syndrome in adolescents. J Pediatr Adolesc Gynecol 20:101–104
32. Mortensen M, Rosenfield RL, Littlejohn E (2006) Functional significance of polycystic-size ovaries in healthy adolescents. J Clin Endocrinol Metab 91:3786–3790
33. Alsamarai S, Adams JM, Murphy MK et al (2009) Criteria for polycystic ovarian morphology in polycystic ovary syndrome as a function for age. J Clin Endocrinol Metab 94:4961–4970
34. Teede HJ, Misso ML, Deeks AA et al (2011) Assessment and management of polycystic ovary syndrome: summary of an evidence-based guideline. Med J Aust 195(6):S65–S112
35. Elting MW, Kwee J, Korsen TJ et al (2003) Aging women with polycystic ovary syndrome who achieve regular menstrual cycles have a smaller follicle cohort than those who continue to have irregular cycles. Fertil Steril 79:1154–1160
36. Bili H, Laven J, Imani B et al (2001) Age-related differences in features associated with polycystic ovary syndrome in normogonadotrophic oligo-amenorrhoeic infertile women of reproductive years. Eur J Endocrinol 145:749–755

37. Murphy MK, Hall JE, Adams JM et al (2006) Polycystic ovarian morphology in normal women does not predict the development of polycystic ovary syndrome. J Clin Endocrinol Metab 91(10):3878–3884
38. Duijkers IJ, Klipping C (2010) Polycystic ovaries, as defined by the 2003 Rotterdam consensus criteria, are found to be very common in young healthy women. Gynecol Endocrinol 26(3):152–160
39. Polson DW, Adams J, Wadsworth J, Franks S (1988) Polycystic ovaries-a common finding in normal women. Lancet 1(8590):870–872
40. Farquhar CM, Birdsall M, Manning P et al (1994) The prevalence of polycystic ovaries on ultrasound scanning in a population of randomly selected women. Aust N Z J Obstet Gynaecol 34(1):67–72
41. Lakhani K, Seifalian AM, Atiomo WU, Hardiman P (2002) Polycystic ovaries. Br J Radiol 75(889):9–16
42. Lujan ME, Jarrett BY, Brooks ED et al (2013) Updated ultrasound criteria for polycystic ovary syndrome: reliable thresholds for elevated follicle population and ovarian volume. Hum Reprod 28(5):1361–1368
43. World Health Organization. STEPwise approach to surveillance (STEPS). Retrieved 21 Mar 2012
44. World Health Organization. Waist circumference and waist-hip ratio. Report of a WHO Expert Consultation. 8–11 Dec 2008. Retrieved 21 Mar 2012
45. Dong Z, Huang J et al (2013) Associations of acanthosis nigricans with metabolic abnormalities in polycystic ovary syndrome women with normal body mass index. J Dermatol 40:188–192
46. de Oliveira R, Penaforte F, Cremonezi Japur C et al (2012) The use of body circumferences for the prediction of intra-abdominal fat in obese women with polycystic ovary syndrome. Nutr Hosp 27(5):1662–1666
47. Callway CW, Chumlea WC, Bouchard C et al (1988) Circumferences. In: Lohman TG, Roche AF, Martorell R (eds) Anthropometric standardization reference manual. Human Kinetics, Champaign, pp 39–54
48. Penaforte FR, Japur CC, Diez-Garcia RW, Chiarello PG (2011) Upper trunk fat assessment and its relationship with metabolic and biochemical variables and body fat in polycystic ovary syndrome. J Hum Nutr Diet 24(1):39–46
49. Dixon JB, O'Brien PE (2002) Neck circumference a good predictor of raised insulin and free androgen index in obese premenopausal women: changes with weight loss. Clin Endocrinol 57:769–778
50. Amato MC, Giordano C, Galia M et al (2010) Visceral adiposity index: a reliable indicator of visceral fat function associated with cardiometabolic risk. Diabetes Care 33:920–922
51. Jee-Young O, Yeon-Ah S, Hye JL (2013) The visceral adiposity index as a predictor of insulin resistance in young women with polycystic ovary syndrome. Obesity 21:1690–1694
52. Macias N, Quezada AD, Flores M et al (2014) Accuracy of body fat percent and adiposity indicators cut off values to detect metabolic risk factors in a sample of Mexican adults. BMC Public Health 14:341
53. Ferland M, Després JP, Tremblay A et al (1989) Assessment of adipose tissue distribution by computed axial tomography in obese women: association with body density and anthropometric measurements. J Nutr 61(2):139–148
54. Jeong Ah K, Chang Jin C, Keun Sang Y (2006) Cut-off values of visceral Fat area and waist circumference: diagnostic criteria for abdominal obesity in a Korean population. J Korean Med Sci 21(6):1048–1053
55. Stoddart ML, Blevins KS, Lee ET et al (2002) Association of acanthosis nigricans with hyperinsulinemia compared with other selected risk factors for type 2 diabetes in Cherokee Indians: the Cherokee Diabetes Study. Diabetes Care 25:1009–1014
56. Kahn CR, Flier JS, Bar RS et al (1976) The syndromes of insulin resistance and acanthosis nigricans insulin-receptor disorders in man. N Engl J Med 294:739–745

57. World Health Organization. Definition, diagnosis and classification of diabetes mellitus and its complications: report of a WHO consultation. Part 1. Diagnosis and classification of diabetes mellitus. Retrieved 29 May 2007
58. Palmert MR, Gordon CM, Kartashov AI et al (2002) Screening for abnormal glucose tolerance in adolescents with polycystic ovary syndrome. J Clin Endocrinol Metab 87(3):1017–1023
59. Wild RA, Carmina E, Diamanti KE et al (2010) Assessment of cardiovascular risk and prevention of cardiovascular disease in women with the polycystic ovary syndrome: a consensus statement by the Androgen Excess and Polycystic Ovary Syndrome (AE-PCOS) Society. J Clin Endocrinol Metab 95:2039–2049
60. Matsuda M, De Fronzo RA (1999) Insulin sensitivity indices obtained from oral glucose tolerance testing: comparison with the euglycemic insulin clamp. Diabetes Care 22:1462–1470
61. Stumvoll M, Van Haeften T et al (2001) Oral glucose tolerance test indexes for insulin sensitivity and secretion based on various availabilities of sampling times. Diabetes Care 24:796–797
62. Matthews DR, Hosker JP et al (1985) Homeostasis model assessment: insulin resistance and beta-cell function from fasting plasma glucose and insulin concentrations in man. Diabetologia 28:412–419
63. Tresaco B, Bueno G, Pineda I et al (2005) Homeostatic model assessment (HOMA) index cut-off values to identify the metabolic syndrome in children. J Physiol Biochem 61(2):381–388
64. Sudhindra MB (2010) Insulin resistance and overweight-obese women with polycystic ovary syndrome. Gynecol Endocrinol 26(5):344–347
65. Legro RS, Finegood D, Dunaif A (1998) A fasting glucose to insulin ratio is a useful measure of insulin sensitivity in women with polycystic ovary syndrome. J Clin Endocrinol Metab 83:2694–2698
66. Veltman-Verhulst S, Goverde AJ et al (2013) Fasting glucose measurement as a potential first step screening for glucose metabolism abnormalities in women with anovulatory polycystic ovary syndrome. Hum Reprod 28:2228–2234
67. Legro RS, Kunselman AR, Dodson WC, Dunaif A (1999) Prevalence and predictors of risk for type 2 diabetes mellitus and impaired glucose tolerance in polycystic ovary syndrome: a prospective, controlled study in 254 affected women. J Clin Endocrinol Metab 84:165–169
68. Lerchbaum E, Schwetz V, Giuliani A et al (2013) Assessment of glucose metabolism in polycystic ovary syndrome: HbA1c or fasting glucose compared with the oral glucose tolerance test as a screening method. Hum Reprod 28(9):2537–2544
69. American Diabetes Association (2012) Standards of medical care in diabetes. Diabetes Care 35(Suppl 1):S11–S63
70. Rizzo M, Longo RA, Guastella E (2011) Assessing cardiovascular risk in mediterranean women with polycystic ovary syndrome. J Endocrinol Invest 34:422–426
71. Bedogni G, Kahn HS, Bellentani S, Tiribelli C (2010) A simple index of lipid overaccumulation is a good marker of liver steatosis. BMC Gastroenterol 10:98
72. Lerchbaum E, Gruber HJ, Schwetz V et al (2011) Fatty liver index in polycystic ovary syndrome. Eur J Endocrinol 165:935–943

PCOS Therapy

6

Gynecologists usually treat PCOS only as an endocrine disorder, without recognition of the very important part that insulin resistance plays in the syndrome.

In this section, the way to treat PCOS from a metabolic point of view, without dwelling on the use of oral contraceptives and antiandrogen drugs, will be discussed.

Lifelong strategies that improve the care of women with PCOS are essential, because of the chronic nature of the syndrome and the young age at which all the symptoms begin to manifest [1].

A valid therapeutic protocol for PCOS includes diet, physical exercise, and insulin-sensitizing agents such as metformin and inositol.

For example, in fact, a normal BMI is associated with a positive fertility outcome, and fertility specialists recommend achieving this BMI before IVF (in vitro fertilization): in fact, these techniques are invasive and expensive and have low success rates, so it seems logical to improve BMI and to support hormonal balance through diet, exercise, and nutrition supplements [2].

6.1 Diet and Exercise

As explained previously, a few evolutionary biologists suppose that many genetic hormonal tendencies contributing to PCOS have their origin in the switch from the pre-agrarian age diet to the current diet. The rapidly increasing rates of diabetes, heart disease, and PCOS coincide with the rapid changes in the modern human diet [2].

All women suffering from PCOS benefit from dietary therapy and exercise; in fact, dietary and lifestyle interventions are considered among the first-line treatments for PCOS.

There is no PCOS diet that will reverse the syndrome, but there are several dietary principles that a patient should follow to improve the symptoms.

© Springer International Publishing Switzerland 2015
M. Stracquadanio, L. Ciotta, *Metabolic Aspects of PCOS: Treatment with Insulin Sensitizers*, DOI 10.1007/978-3-319-16760-2_6

Weight reduction leads to improvements of insulin sensitivity [3] and lipid profile [4]; it ameliorates hyperandrogenism (SHBG increase, FAI and testosterone decrease) and menstrual cycle rhythm [4–6], with reductions in adiposity from the truncal–abdominal area [5]. Moreover, there is evidence that these changes exert important beneficial effects also in the longer term on disorders such as type II diabetes mellitus, cardiovascular disease, and certain cancers (endometrial, breast, and colon cancer), compared with weight loss alone [7–9].

In most of the dietary studies in women with PCOS, improvements in metabolic and reproductive outcomes have been closely related to improvements in insulin sensitivity, suggesting that dietary modification (qualitative and quantitative) designed to improve insulin resistance may produce greater benefits than those achieved by energy restriction alone [7].

Clinicians prescribing lifestyle modifications must consider the patient's capacity to sustain diet and exercise adherence and weight maintenance over time for the clinical benefits on PCOS to continue.

Considering how difficult it is for many patients to change their lifestyle, pharmaceutical modification of weight control could be an additional necessary therapeutic tool, such as the lipase inhibitor orlistat [10].

In some studies on overweight and obese women with PCOS, the use of orlistat has demonstrated an improvement in both metabolic and hormonal parameters [11, 12].

Orlistat is an antiobesity drug with minimal systemic absorption, and therefore, any effect of this drug is a result of weight loss and not the direct effect on ovaries.

The proposal therapeutic dose is 120 mg three times daily, before each meal, for 3 months, during which the patient must be able to lose at least 5 % of its total weight.

6.1.1   PCOS Dietary Recommendations

1. *Reduce total calories consumed to standard levels for sex, age, and activity*: calories requests are higher for women with higher BMI and increase in relation to activity. It is often useful to initially focus on the eating pattern and the macronutrient content of the diet rather than to try to promote both healthy eating and weight loss too quickly [8]. Energy consumption can be reached by limiting nutrient intake or by increasing calories expenditure.

   A daily calories deficit of 200 kcal/day will prevent weight gain; a deficit of 500 kcal/day is needed for the average person to lose 0.5 kg/week, while a 1,000 kcal deficit is needed for 1 kg weight loss/week [8].

2. *Reduce refined carbohydrates in favor of complex carbohydrates.* "Refined" carbohydrates refer to a carbohydrate-based food that has been processed to strip it of some of its original fiber and unpackaged to produce a more "refined" product. For example, sugar cane and corn on the cob are whole foods, but the table sugar that is processed out of sugar cane and the cornstarch or high fructose corn syrup processed out of the corn are some refined carbohydrates [2].

A period of relatively strict carbohydrate restriction helps at the beginning of the diet; a recent study demonstrated that a reduced-carbohydrate diet results in lower measures of β-cell responsiveness and circulating insulin (27 % reduction in fasting insulin) when compared with a standard higher-carbohydrate diet [13].

Other studies have reported improvements in LDL cholesterol particle size, LDL concentration, and postprandial blood lipid profile [14–16].

On the other hand, low-carbohydrate diets have been associated with deleterious effects on lipid profile when used long term [17], and so severe carbohydrate restriction should be use as a short-term measure to achieve weight loss [8].

3. *Eat low-glycemic index (GI) foods*: a few studies have shown that a low-GI diet can improve insulin resistance as well as many of its metabolic consequences including increasing HDL and plasminogen activator inhibitor-1 levels [18, 19]. Moreover, several epidemiological studies have also associated a low-GI diet with reduced risk of CVD and type II diabetes [20, 21].

   A high-GI diet, on the other hand, has been shown to worsen postprandial insulin resistance [22]: in fact, a recent study showed that a low-GI diet improves insulin sensitivity and menstrual regularity more than a conventional healthy, moderate- to high-GI diet despite similar weight loss [23].

4. *Increase fiber to improve glucose regulation*: fiber helps to slow the digestion of carbohydrates and improves insulin resistance [24, 25].

5. *Increase high-protein foods*: it was demonstrated that proteins consumed at breakfast (compared with lunch or dinner) lead to a greater initial and sustained feeling of fullness, increased satiety, and reduced concentrations of the appetite-regulating hormone ghrelin [26–28].

   Adequate protein intake is important to protect lean body mass and to increase muscle in response to exercise [8]. Actually, there is little evidence to suggest benefits of high-protein diets on insulin resistance, and a number of studies in women with PCOS have failed to show significant long-term benefits of a high-protein diet on weight loss or insulin sensitivity [16, 29]; there are also concerns about the safety of high-protein, low-carbohydrate diets including the effects of kidney function and bone mineral density [7].

6. *Increase food rich in omega-3 essential fatty acids (PUFAs)*: they have an important role in human cell metabolism; an US study investigated the positive effects of a polyunsaturated fatty acid (PUFA)-rich diet in PCOS patients [28], but further research is required to determine real beneficial and harmful effects of various PUFAs in insulin-resistant populations.

7. *Meal timing*: the frequency and regularity of eating patterns are important, even if there are small data in the literature.

   One of the largest studies [29] conducted revealed that those who ate frequently during the day had higher intakes of carbohydrates, fibers, and a range of micronutrients, while those who ate less frequently had higher intakes of fat, cholesterol, protein, and sodium.

   Other studies showed that a regular meal frequency leads to higher postprandial energy expenditure, lower energy intake, and improved impaired insulin sensitivity compared with irregular eating in 2-week interventions

[30]. In a further study, breakfast consumption was associated with a lower energy intake and improved insulin sensitivity compared with breakfast omission [31].

Data in literature show that a diet with 50 % of total calories from carbohydrates (with a low glycemic index), 30 % from fat (mostly mono- and polyunsaturated fat, less than 10 % from saturated fat), 20 % from proteins, and high in fiber is the most appropriate for patients with PCOS [32].

The optimal frequency of food intake has yet to be determined: however, a regular pattern with low intake from snacks is advisable [8], and high-calorie intake at breakfast with reduced intake at dinner is suggested, because it leads to reduced overall insulin levels [33–35].

6.1.2 Glycemic Index (GI)

It has been shown that eating foods with a low GI improves glucose control in women with PCOS and diabetes.

The glycemic index indicates the rate in which glycemia increases after taking a quantity of "X" food containing 50 g of carbohydrates.

Foods with carbohydrates that break down quickly during digestion and release glucose rapidly into the bloodstream tend to have a high GI; foods with carbohydrates that break down more slowly, emitting glucose more gradually into the bloodstream, tend to have a low GI [2].

The concept was developed by Dr. David J. Jenkins and colleagues [36] in 1980–1981 at the University of Toronto in their research to find out which foods were best for people with diabetes. A lower glycemic index suggests slower rates of digestion and absorption of the foods' carbohydrates and may also indicate greater extraction from the liver and periphery of the products of carbohydrate digestion.

A lower glycemic response usually relates to a lower insulin demand but not always and may improve long-term blood glucose control and blood lipids [37]. The glycemic index of a food is defined as the incremental area under the 2-h blood glucose response curve (AUC) following a 12-h fast and ingestion of a food with a certain quantity of available carbohydrate (usually 50 g). The AUC of the test food is divided by the AUC of the standard (either glucose or white bread, giving two different definitions) and multiplied by 100. The average GI value is calculated from data collected in ten human subjects. Both the standard and test food must contain an equal amount of available carbohydrate. The result gives a relative ranking for each tested food [38]. The GI Symbol Program is an independent worldwide GI certification program that helps consumers identify low-GI foods and drinks. The symbol is only on foods or beverages that have had their GI values tested according to the standard and meet the GI Foundation's certification criteria as a healthy choice within their food group. GI cutoffs are listed in Table 6.1.

Table 6.1 Glycemic index cutoffs

Glycemic index cutoffs	
High	≥70
Moderate	50–70
Low	<50

Of course, the glycemic index has also its limitations: the index calculations are not accurate because the behavior of foods in different individuals can change, and judging the diet by GI alone does not give the whole portrait of the diet [2].

Moreover, GI values depend on how foods are cooked: cooked carrots have a higher GI than raw carrots because cooking breaks down the fiber and the glucose can be absorbed much more quickly. Cooking with a bit of salt or vinegar may lower the GI of many vegetables because this causes many molecules, not just the sugars, to be broken down, which results in trapping some of the starches in complex structures that are digested more slowly [2].

Furthermore, for some people, a food consumed in the morning on an empty stomach will spike the blood sugar more than the same food eaten later in the day after having breakfast: patients with good blood sugar control in general will show less of a spike in blood sugar than someone with poor blood sugar control [2].

PCOS women should follow some useful GI advices for their daily diet:

- *Eat five to ten different whole fresh fruits, vegetables, and legumes each day.*
- *Avoid a diet that consists predominantly of the food highest on the glycemic index.*
- *Substitute foods high on the GI with foods lower on the GI*: for example, eat boiled green beans (GI of 15) instead of boiled potatoes (GI of 100) with dinner (Table 6.2).
- *Increase fiber intake*: fiber helps to slow the digestion of carbohydrates and improves insulin resistance. If a food high on the GI is loved, patient should take care not to consume it often and aim to eat only a small portion of it combined with high-fiber foods that reduce the glycemic index [24, 25].
- *Eat legumes to lower the high-GI foods in the meals*: legumes are low on the GI and contain an impressive amount of fiber and good-quality protein, which can serve to blunt the glycemic load. Moreover, legumes contain pinitol, a relative of D-chiro-inositol, noted for improving insulin resistance [2].
- *Avoid overeating foods high on the glycemic index.* The GI of a food can be tempered by the quantity consumed. For example, a piece of candy might have a very high glycemic index, but eating just one little piece will not result in a high glycemic load on the body; if the patient eats two pieces of white toast, jam, brown potatoes, and a sugar- or corn syrup-sweetened fruit drink for breakfast, she is putting a high glycemic load on her body, and the blood sugar will remain high for several hours as her body works to process the large amount of high-GI foods [2].
- *Evaluate the whole meat, rather than individual food items*, to make sure the patient is preparing meals that will not spike her blood sugars.

Table 6.2 Foods' glycemic index list

Foods' glycemic index	
Sweeteners	
Corn syrup	100
Table sugar (sucrose)	100
Rice syrup	65
Honey	54
Fructose	10
Stevia	0
Grains	
White rice	90
Rice cakes	84
Wild rice	81
Corn chips	72
Cornmeal	70
Couscous	65
Brown rice	55
Pop corn	55
Whole wheat	48
Whole amaranth	35
Bread	
Rice bread	100
Polenta	98
Baguettes	95
Doughnuts	76
Croissant	70
White bread	70
Pancakes	67
Kamut bread	54
Rye bread	50
Pasta, whole grain	44
Wheat germ	15
Cereals	
Instant oats	92
Puffed rice	85
Grape-Nuts	67
Oat bran	15
Nuts and seeds	
Chestnuts	60
Peanut butter	40
Sesame seeds	35
Almonds	15
Hazelnuts	15
Pistachios	14

Table 6.2 (continued)

Foods' glycemic index	
Walnuts	14
Peanuts	14
Legumes and beans	
Fava beans	50
Black beans	35
Hummus	35
White beans	35
Lentils	29
Soybeans	18
Green beans	15
Tofu	14
Vegetables	
Potatoes, baked	100
Potatoes, boiled	84
Carrots, cooked	80
Beets, cooked	64
Corn	55
Peas	44
Coconut	35
Tomato sauce	35
Carrots, raw	30
Asparagus	15
Cucumbers	15
Lettuce	15
Mushrooms	15
Olives	15
Spinach	15
Tomatoes	15
Zucchini	15
Avocados	10
Fruits	
Watermelons	90
Pineapples	66
Apricots	57
Strawberries	56
Mangos	55
Bananas	52
Grapes	50
Oranges	46
Apples	39
Peaches	30
Raspberries	25

(continued)

Table 6.2 (continued)

Foods' glycemic index	
Cherries	25
Others	
Beer	110
Rice milk	84
Mango juice	55
Orange juice	45
Coconut milk	40
Soy milk	36
Yogurt, low-fat fruit	33
Almond milk	30
Dark chocolate	25
Lemon juice	20
Pesto	15
Vinegar	5
Water	0

6.1.3   Glycemic Load (GL)

Some authors believe that the glycemic load (GL) is a more useful measure of food value than the glycemic index alone.

Glycemic load accounts for how much carbohydrate is in the food and how much each gram of carbohydrate in the food raises blood glucose levels.

GL is a GI-weighted measure of carbohydrate content [39].

$$GL = GI \times carbohydrate\,(grams)\,/\,100$$

For instance, watermelon has a high GI, but a typical portion of watermelon does not contain many carbohydrates, so the glycemic load of eating it is low. Whereas glycemic index is defined for each type of food, glycemic load can be calculated for any size serving of a food, an entire meal, or an entire day's meals.

GL cutoffs are listed in Table 6.3.

Foods that have a low GL in a typical serving size have usually a low GI. Foods with an intermediate or high GL in a typical serving size range from a very low to very high GI (Table 6.4).

For detailed information about all the foods, visit the website www.glycemicindex.com

Table 6.3 Glycemic load cutoffs

Glycemic load cutoffs	
High	$\geq$20
Intermediate	11–19
Low	<10

Table 6.4 Foods' glycemic load list

Glycemic load (per 100 g serving)	
Baguette	15
Banana	16
Potato	20
Carrots	2
Rice	30
Watermelon	4

6.1.4 Insulin Index

The insulin index is a measure used to quantify the typical insulin response to various foods. The index is similar to the glycemic index and glycemic load, but rather than relying on glycemia levels, the insulin index is based upon insulinemia. This measure can be more useful than either the glycemic index or the glycemic load because certain foods (e.g., lean meats and proteins) cause an insulin response despite there being no carbohydrates present, and some foods cause a disproportionate insulin response relative to their carbohydrate load [40].

Holt et al. have noted that the glucose and insulin scores of most foods are highly correlated, but high-protein foods and bakery products that are rich in fat and refined carbohydrates "elicit insulin responses that were disproportionately higher than their glycemic responses" [40]. They also conclude that insulin indices may be useful for dietary management and avoidance of non-insulin-dependent diabetes mellitus and hyperlipidemia.

Glycemic Index (GI) considers each food relative to eating 100 % glucose, while the insulin index is relative to eating white bread (GI of ~70 to 75) (Table 6.5).

6.1.5 Exercise

Exercise reduces insulin resistance by two mechanisms. It induces a reduction in visceral fat even if it results in moderate weight loss and BMI reduction [41]. Visceral fat is more metabolically active than subcutaneous fat and central adiposity is more closely related to IR [32].

Exercise, besides, increases muscle cell metabolism: it modulates the expression or the activity of proteins mediating insulin signaling in the skeletal muscles [41, 42].

It has been shown that exercise improves menstrual abnormalities and restores ovulation in obese patients with PCOS [43], and its benefit on reproductive function is greater than the benefit of low-calories diet only [44].

Exercise exerts its beneficial effects on body composition with a 45 % greater reduction in fat mass and a 60 % better preservation of fat-free mass [45].

In fact, it is important to clarify that improved abdominal obesity and insulin sensitivity may occur without a total change in body weight: body composition of

Table 6.5 Foods' glycemic and insulin index list

	Glycemic index	Insulin index
Porridge	60±12	40±4
Muesli	43±7	46±5
Cornflakes	76±11	75±8
Average:	59±3	57±3
White bread (baseline)	71±0	100±0
White pasta	46±10	40±5
Brown pasta	68±10	40±5
Brown rice	104±18	62±11
French fries	71±16	74±12
White rice	110±15	79±12
Whole-meal bread	97±17	96±12
Potatoes	141±35	121±11
Eggs	42±16	31±6
Cheese	55±18	45±13
Beef	21±8	51±16
Lentils	62±22	58±12

patients who exercise regularly may change with increased lean body mass and decreased fat mass, but no overall change in weight [8].

At the moment, there are no guidelines for the type, intensity, frequency, and duration of exercise in patients with PCOS [45, 46].

6.1.5.1 PCOS Exercise Recommendations

1. Moderate-intensity aerobic physical activity (e.g., brisk walking) for at least 30 min and for at least 5 days per week should be recommended in all PCOS patients [32].
2. Vigorous-intensity aerobic activity (e.g., jogging) for at least 20 min and for at least 3 days per week or combinations of moderate- and vigorous-intensity exercise can also be recommended [32].
3. Resistance training for at least two nonconsecutive days per week [32].
4. Endurance exercise: for patients who cannot manage high-intensity exercise, prolonged lower-level activity is an appropriate way to gain fitness and to increase energy expenditure [8].

6.2 Insulin-Sensitizing Agents and Statins

Examining scientific literature, studies are very conflicting to each other, and a unanimous opinion on the effectiveness of insulin-sensitizing drugs has not yet been reached.

According to the ASRM Committee of 2008, insulin-sensitizing agents should be considered in patients with impaired glucose tolerance (IGT) and PCOS [47].

Particularly, in 2010, AE-PCOS Society consensus treatment emphasized that metformin should be used in women with PCOS who have already started lifestyle treatment (diet and exercise) and do not have improvement in IGT or in those who have normal weight but still having IGT [48].

When administered to insulin-resistant patients, these drugs act to increase target tissue responsiveness in order to reduce hyperinsulinemia [49].

In the past, limited studies on the use of diazoxide, acarbose, and somatostatin for PCOS women were conducted; then, thiazolidinediones aroused more interest, while, to date, metformin is the most worldwide studied insulin-sensitizing agent.

Moreover, statins have also been used to improve lipid profile in PCOS women.

6.2.1   Thiazolidinediones

Thiazolidinediones (TZDs) include pioglitazone, rosiglitazone, and troglitazone: during the past, they have been used in PCOS women to reduce insulin resistance.

TZDs are selective ligands of the nuclear transcription factor peroxisome proliferator-activated receptor-γ (PPAR-γ) [50].

They exert their insulin-sensitizing actions by two mechanisms:

- Promoting fatty acid uptake and storage in adipose tissue
- Increasing the expression of adiponectin, an adipocytokine with an insulin sensitivity effect [51]

Obese women with PCOS who were administered troglitazone demonstrated benefit in insulin sensitivity, glucose tolerance, and hyperandrogenemia [52–56].

It was demonstrated that even pioglitazone, in doses of 30 mg/day for 3 months, significantly improved insulin sensitivity, hyperandrogenism, and ovulation rates [56].

TZDs were shown to be more effective than metformin in reducing levels of free testosterone and DHEAS after 3 months of treatment, but this benefit was not evident after 6 months of therapy [57].

Pioglitazone is able to produce a significant reduction in the incidence of impaired glucose tolerance and 40 % reversion of previous IGT to normal in PCOS patients treated with 45 mg daily for 6 months [58]. Significant improvements of insulin effectiveness in the liver and skeletal muscle, with substantial increase of circulating adiponectin levels, were also reported [59].

Moreover, some studies demonstrated a clear capacity of pioglitazone to reduce free fatty acid level in PCOS patients, by decreasing lipolysis and increasing lipogenesis [60]; conversely, other studies failed to show any improvement in lipid profile [61].

Additionally, some studies indicate a reduction of inflammatory markers in pioglitazone-treated PCOS women [62], while others do not [58].

A randomized study using treatment with pioglitazone showed that the latter increased ovulation frequency [63]. The regulation of ovulation could in turn restore normal feedback effects of luteal steroids, normalize serum LH levels, and improve ovarian steroidogenesis [64]. Additionally, pioglitazone was shown to ameliorate GnRH-stimulated LH secretion [56].

Administration of pioglitazone during ovarian stimulation period seems to improve ovarian response to controlled ovarian stimulation in PCOS patients, in terms of clinical pregnancy rate, as well as risks of ovarian hyperstimulation syndrome and multiple pregnancies [64].

Previously, TZDs have been accused of inducing weight gain and water retention, but recent studies have disconfirmed this supposition [65].

However, the primary concern with TZDs is the liver toxicity: a significant number of cases of hepatic necrosis were reported in patients using troglitazone, which was withdrawn from the market in 2000.

Pioglitazone safety in women under 18 is not yet established, so it is not recommended in this female PCOS subgroup.

However, in clinical practice, neither pioglitazone nor rosiglitazone is routinely used in PCOS women, especially with infertility issues, because TZDs are classified as pregnancy category C by the FDA, due to the fact that studies in animals have shown adverse fetal effects such as IUGR [64].

6.2.2 Metformin

Despite there is no universal consensus on metformin benefits in PCOS, in this chapter all the beneficial effects of metformin therapy in patients with PCOS are highlighted.

The positive effects of metformin have been demonstrated in nondiabetic women with PCOS, and they are associated with increased menstrual cyclicity, improved ovulation, and reduction in circulating androgen levels [66].

To date neither in Europe nor in the United States metformin has been approved for the treatment of insulin resistance associated with PCOS: its use should be restricted to those patients with IGT [67]; however, it is largely prescribed as an "off-label" drug.

For "off-label" use of any medication, it is extremely important to fulfill several criteria for safe use:

- The condition should have health consequences significant enough to warrant treatment.
- The treatment should have demonstrated safety and efficacy.
- The proposed treatment should be superior to the presently available alternatives [68].

6.2.2.1 Mechanism of Action

Metformin is a second-generation biguanide used as an oral antihyperglycemic agent, and it is approved by the US Food and Drug Administration (FDA) as treatment for type II diabetes mellitus.

It is considered an insulin-sensitizing agent because it lowers glucose levels without increasing insulin secretion, but improving insulin sensitivity.

Metformin causes [69, 70]:

- Increased peripheral insulin sensitivity, by activating glucose transporters (GLUTs) which allows passage of glucose into hepatic and muscle cells
- Inhibition of hepatic glucose production
- Reduction of circulating free fatty acid concentrations, which helps in reducing gluconeogenesis

Metformin activates the adenosine monophosphate (AMP)-activated protein kinase pathway (AMPK) [71, 72]: phosphorylation of threonine in AMPK is necessary for metformin action, resulting in decreased glucose production and increased fatty acid oxidation in hepatocytes, skeletal muscle cells [73], and mouse ovarian tissue [74].

Furthermore, metformin inhibits hepatic gluconeogenesis through an AMP-activated protein kinase-dependent regulation of the orphan nuclear receptor small heterodimer partner (SHP) [75, 76].

Importantly, the actions of metformin are not associated with an increase in insulin secretion and, consequently, with hypoglycemia.

Metformin affects ovarian function in a dual mode:

- Alleviation of systemic insulin excess acting upon the ovary, particularly on steroidogenesis and follicular growth
- Direct ovarian effect

Furthermore, metformin acts at the hypothalamic level on AMPK pathway: the latter is essential in the modulation of LH secretion [77].

During the last two decades, some studies demonstrated that metformin inhibits androstenedione and testosterone production from theca cells through inhibition of the steroidogenic acute regulatory protein and 17α-hydroxylase expression [78].

At the ovarian level, hyperandrogenic intrafollicular pattern is improved by a decrease in IGF-1 availability that has an important role in controlling granulosa cell aromatase levels [79].

It has been shown that granulosa cells from women with PCOS have higher levels of FSH receptor (FSHR) expression compared with those from normal ovaries [80, 81].

Metformin reduces FSH-stimulated aromatase expression and activity in granulosa cells; it exerts this action by reducing FSHR mRNA and consequently the activity of FSH (as measured by aromatase expression and E_2), without altering cAMP levels. This involves blocking activation of CRE on promoter II of CYP19 via inhibition of pCREB and possible disruption of the formation of the CREB-CRTC2 co-activator complex. This is via an AMPK-independent mechanism [82].

6.2.2.2 Dosage and Side Effects

Metformin is available as 500, 850, and 1,000 mg tablets with a target dose of 1,500–2,550 mg/day.

Metformin has a dose-dependent absorption in humans [83], and its bioavailability is limited to 50–60 % because the amount available may result from pre-systemic clearance or binding to the intestinal wall [83].

Therapeutic regimens of metformin administration are not well standardized, and its dose should probably be adjusted according to the patient's BMI and insulin resistance [84].

For example, it was demonstrated that nonobese women with PCOS respond better than obese women to metformin treatment at a dosage of 1,500 mg/day for 6 months. Nonobese women, in fact, showed a statistically significant decrease in serum androgen level and fasting insulin level and also an improvement in menstrual cyclicity [85, 86]. Moreover, it is possible that women who did not respond to metformin 1,5 g dose per day might show clinical changes if the dose is increased to 2 g [76].

Common side effects are gastrointestinal, such as diarrhea, nausea, vomiting, bloating, abdominal discomfort, flatulence, and unpleasant metallic taste in the mouth.

Lactic acidosis and hypoglycemia are very rare.

To reduce these side effects, it is recommended to start metformin with a low dose (e.g., 250–500 mg/day) and then gradually increase within a period of 4–6 weeks [76].

Metformin may cause vitamin B12 malabsorption, and so every patient should be monitored for signs and symptoms of vitamin B12 deficiency: numbness, paresthesia, macroglossia, behavioral changes, and pernicious anemia [66].

Metformin prescription should be avoided in women with renal insufficiency, congestive heart failure, sepsis, or hepatic dysfunction [66].

Therefore, testing of hepatic and renal function is necessary in advance of prescription, and thereafter yearly testing is indicated.

However, it has been demonstrated that metformin use for up to 6 months does not adversely affect renal or liver function in a large sample of PCOS women, even those with mildly abnormal baseline hepatic parameters [87, 88].

The length of metformin treatment in PCOS patients is not standardized, but data present in literature [89] showed that, after a long-term metformin treatment, drug suspension is related to a quick reversion of its beneficial effect on peripheral insulin sensitivity.

6.2.2.3   Metformin and Menstrual Disorders

The main complaint about menstrual disorders from PCOS patients is the absence or infrequency of menstrual bleeding.

Few studies noticed the regularization of menstrual cycle after 3–6 months of therapy with metformin alone in 60–70 % of PCOS insulin-resistant patients [90–93] with an important improvement of LH/FSH ratio [90].

The response to the treatment usually depends on the degree of insulin resistance.

The positive effect of metformin on menstrual cycle is commonly attributed to its effectiveness on ovulatory function. However, it is not uncommon to observe discordance between menstrual and ovulatory cycles.

The presence of ovulation should be confirmed through the measurement of luteal phase progesterone levels (usually, levels > 4 ng/mL indicate a previous ovulation) [76].

An Italian study revealed that only 79 % of PCOS women had ovulatory cycles after reaching normal menstrual cycle with metformin treatment [93].

This observation may indicate that the effectiveness of metformin on menstrual cyclicity is probably secondary to a direct effect on the endometrium and not only to an effect on the ovary [67].

Ovulation may be a result of a direct action of metformin on the ovary that leads to normal steroid production and steroid feedback effects that include a lowering of LH and androgen levels [67].

6.2.2.4 Metformin and Endometrium

Excessive insulin levels stimulate endometrial growth [94], and most anovulatory PCOS patients have endometrial vascularization and pattern and thickness abnormalities [95, 96]: PI (pulsatility index) and RI (resistance index) are higher than controls, probably due to the vasoconstrictive effect of androgens on vascular tissues [97].

Metformin may have a positive impact on the endometrium thanks to:

- Indirect effect: androgen decrease, which leads to the reduction of their vasoconstrictive effects on vascular tissue.
- Direct effect: insulin stimulates glucose oxidation activity in the late luteal phase in human endometrium; insulin receptors are present at the endometrial level, reaching their maximal expression in the secretory phase. GLUT-4 is an insulin-dependent transporter expressed in the endometrium and involved in endometrium metabolism; GLUT-4 is reduced in PCOS patients, suggesting that in these subjects both insulin resistance and hyperinsulinemia induce an inadequate GLUT-4 expression and so a decreased glucose supply. Thus, by improving hyperinsulinemia, metformin could be effective in restoring endometrial receptivity through a direct effect.

PCOS women who ovulated under metformin treatment showed a triple-line endometrial pattern in a percentage of cases similar to those observed in healthy controls [95], and a triple-line pattern is associated with a significantly higher pregnancy rate.

Another aim of metformin treatment is to reduce the long-term risks of unchallenged endometrial proliferation: hyperplasia and carcinoma.

Their main pathogenic mechanism assumed was hyper-estrogenic stimulation of endometrial growth, unopposed by progesterone. In fact, estrogens act by genetic and epigenetic mechanisms on cancer cells, and a close relationship between estrogens, growth factors, and oncogenes is important in the development of several human cancer [98].

The second hypothesis taken in consideration was the known mitogenic effect exerted by insulin [99].

6.2.2.5 Metformin and Hyperandrogenism

Metformin determines a great improvement on the hyperandrogenism symptoms of patients with PCOS, ameliorating hyperandrogenemia and reducing circulating insulin levels [92, 101–103]. Moreover, as insulin acts as an anabolic growth factor in hair [104], it is possible that the suppression of circulating insulin levels alone may be sufficient to improve the rate of terminal hair growth [76].

A 20–30 % reduction of total and free testosterone, increased SHBG levels, a 30 % decline of androstenedione levels, a modest decrease of FG hirsutism score, and an improvement of acanthosis nigricans were shown [92, 100].

Poor effects on the acne score of young PCOS women were recorded [105].

Several data suggest that metformin could act on hyperandrogenism by interfering both with direct and specific mechanisms on peripheral androgen-secreting organs and with free androgen fraction-regulating systems [67]: in fact, a reduced ovarian and adrenal secretion of androgens, a reduced pituitary secretion of LH, and an increased liver SHBG production seem to be the mechanisms that mediate metformin effect on hyperandrogenism [69].

On the other hand, other studies compared metformin effects to those obtained from oral contraceptives or antiandrogen drugs: the latter achieved a more effective results on hyperandrogenism than metformin alone [106–108].

According to our clinical experience, in overweight/insulin-resistant/hirsute PCOS women, metformin should be considered a first-line treatment, to be associated in combination with antiandrogen therapy.

Moreover, a case reported by an English study group demonstrated how important is the metformin administration even in underweight PCOS patients with menstrual disorder and hirsutism, underlying the essential role of insulin resistance in PCOS pathogenesis, sometimes independent of fat mass or distribution [109].

6.2.2.6 Metformin and Fertility

Metformin reduces insulin levels and alters its effects on ovarian androgen biosynthesis, theca cell proliferation, and endometrial growth; it inhibits ovarian gluconeogenesis, reducing ovarian androgen production [110–112]: all these actions lead to an improved ovulation induction in PCOS patients.

According to the ESHRE and ASRM guidelines issued in 2007, the use of metformin should be limited to patients with impaired glucose tolerance and should be interrupted before the administration of clomiphene citrate, thus restricting the use of metformin to a minority of PCOS patients [113].

However, more recent data suggest that these guidelines should be reconsidered.

Metformin alone has a significant benefit on inducing ovulation in PCOS women, but there is limited evidence that it improves pregnancy rate [101]. According to a multicenter study, metformin alone is not as effective as clomiphene citrate (CC) alone for the treatment of infertility: 55.3 vs. 75.1 % in cumulative ovulation and 7.2 % vs. 22.5 % of life birth [101].

On the contrary, an Italian study stated that the cumulative ovulation rate was similar in women treated with CC or metformin, whereas the pregnancy rate was significantly higher in women treated with metformin [114].

However, metformin is more effective than placebo alone, and it is associated with a significantly lower multiple pregnancy and ovarian hyperstimulation syndrome (OHSS) rate [76].

Because of the lack of evidence, metformin should not be used as first-line monotherapy, but only in those patients who:

1. Want to improve both metabolic and reproductive functions, but they do not want to immediately get pregnant.
2. Absolutely wish to avoid multiple gestations.
3. Do not tolerate CC or are resistant to CC [76].
    Clomiphene resistance is defined as the inability to achieve ovulation after two cycles of clomiphene administration at a dose of 150 mg/day for 5 days [115].
4. Do not achieve a pregnancy (CC failure): metformin could be administered as pretreatment [67].

In CC-resistant women, a combined therapy with CC + metformin (contemporarily or as pretreatment) is suggested: in a meta-analysis, this combination significantly improved ovulation and pregnancy rates, decreasing OHSS rate, when compared with CC alone [116].

The percentage of patients with PCOS and clomiphene resistance ranges in the different studies between 15 and 40 % [117, 118]. In these patients, metformin/clomiphene combination induces ovulation in 62.5–77.7 % of cases [116, 119–122].

This result is probably secondary to various mechanisms:

- Changes in intrafollicular steroidogenesis resulting from the effect of metformin on granulosa cells through an increase in insulin-like growth factor 1 [120]
- Inhibition of androgen synthesis by the direct action of metformin on the interna theca cells [78]
- Metformin-induced decrease of adrenal responsiveness to adrenocorticotropic hormone, resulting in reduced adrenal steroidogenesis [123]
- Reduction in serum LH and prolactin levels resulting from the effects of metformin on the hypothalamic–pituitary axis [124]

Thus, it is possible to state that metformin administration, decreasing insulin secretion, facilitates the induction of ovulation by using clomiphene citrate [125] in patients with PCOS.

The beneficial effects of metformin coadministration during gonadotropin ovulation induction and/or IVF cycles are unclear, and therapy with metformin should depend on the degree of IR.

It is well known that the response of PCOS women to gonadotropin stimulation differs significantly from that of normal ovaries: it is defined "explosive" and it is responsible for the higher risk of canceled cycles and/or for OHSS [126, 127].

In fact, it was shown that during ovarian stimulation, E_2 production and E_2-to-A ratio are higher in patients with PCOS who have elevated insulin levels than in normo-insulinemic women [126]. Increased insulin levels involve greater ovarian endocrine and morphologic responses to FSH-induced ovulation, which predispose to OHSS.

Therefore, it seems that the typical response of the polycystic ovary to exogenous gonadotropin therapy is related to increased plasma concentrations of insulin [128].

6.2.2.7 Metformin and Pregnancy Loss

Few observational studies have shown that metformin could play an important role in reducing the risk of pregnancy loss [129–131].

In particular, metformin exerts systemic actions by reducing body weight, insulin and PAI-1 levels [131–133], and plasmatic endothelin-1 (ET-1), androgen, and LH concentrations [135] and by increasing IGFBP-1 and glycodelin levels [136].

Moreover, metformin improved the uterine artery blood flow [95, 136] and several endometrial receptivity surrogate markers, as well as endometrial vascularization and pattern [95]. It was hypothesized that metformin might improve perifollicular and peri-corpus luteum vascularization too [95].

Furthermore, in the past, an experimental study [137] demonstrated that metformin also induced AMPK activation within the blastocyst, leading to improved insulin signaling and pregnancy outcomes. In fact, the preimplantation blastocyst stage embryo is an insulin-sensitive tissue, responsive to insulin or IGF-1 via the IGF-1 receptor/translocation of GLUT-4, with an increased glucose uptake [138]. High insulin or IGF-1 concentrations induced a downregulation of IGF-1 receptor [139] with consequent insulin-stimulated glucose uptake reduction, intraembryonic glucose level dropping, and apoptosis triggering [138].

On the contrary, other studies did not confirm these beneficial effects of metformin in preventing abortion [140, 141].

6.2.2.8 Metformin Administration During Pregnancy

The safety of metformin in pregnancy has not yet been established. It crosses the human placenta [142, 143], and it has been detected in umbilical cord blood at levels equal to or higher than the ones in maternal venous blood [144–146]: in fact, except for the first hours after metformin intake, the fetus is exposed to higher concentrations of metformin than the mother [144]. The knowledge on metformin metabolism in the fetus is scarce: it has been hypothesized that part of the metformin is excreted to the amniotic fluid [147] and reabsorbed to the fetal circulation by swallowing. Metformin is then eliminated from the fetus by passage through the placenta into the maternal circulation [144]. Fetal insulin concentrations are not affected by maternal metformin treatment.

A recent study demonstrated that intrauterine metformin exposure seems to result in elevated SHBG levels in newborns [148]. Metformin exposure throughout pregnancy exerts no major effects on maternal or neonatal androgens or estrogens at birth [148].

Metformin is classified as pregnancy category B [149]: a meta-analysis concluded that there was no evidence of an increased risk for major malformations [150].

Additionally, a study demonstrated that metformin did not adversely affect birth length, birth weight, growth, or motor–social development in the first 18 months of life [151].

However, current conservative practice would be to stop treatment once pregnancy has been established, but considering the adverse impact of insulin resistance on the pregnancy, continued metformin treatment after conception in women with PCOS may be beneficial [152].

The rationale of using metformin during pregnancy in PCOS women is the attempt to reduce the risk of developing gestational diabetes and other pregnancy complications associated with insulin resistance, such as preeclampsia.

Metformin seems to reduce the risk of gestational diabetes (GD) [153, 154] that complicates 5–40 % of pregnancy in women with PCOS.

Continued metformin treatment throughout pregnancy appeared to significantly reduce the rate of GDM requiring insulin therapy [155].

The mechanisms recognized in reducing GD incidence were the reduction of preconception weight, insulin, insulin resistance, insulin secretion, and testosterone levels and the persistence of these effects during pregnancy [156].

A less weight gain in women treated with metformin, compared with those treated with insulin, has been reported, and also the incidence of neonatal hypoglycemia was reduced [157, 158].

Furthermore, during the first trimester of pregnancy, metformin seems to influence the trophoblastic invasion of the maternal decidua, myometrium, and blood vessels, allowing a successful placentation with consequent pregnancy outcome improvement, such as prevention of pregnancy-induced hypertension (PIH) and preeclampsia [67].

Increased placental insulin resistance directly impairs nutrient supply to the fetus and leads to fetal growth restriction [159, 160].

Unfortunately, there are only a few studies in literature confirming these preliminary data.

Generally, it is important to note that the beneficial role of metformin in pregnancy-related parameters may be accomplished through a continuum of effects that starts from preconception and lasts throughout pregnancy [152]. In fact, preconception weight loss and IR reduction promoted by the combination of metformin and diet may reduce the likelihood of gestational diabetes in PCOS women [156].

Despite these favorable effects and reassuring clinical data, no definite guidelines recommending metformin use in pregnant women exist: further research is necessary [157, 161].

Finally, it is important to know that metformin is transferred into breast milk in amounts that appear to be clinically insignificant [162–165]. Thus, metformin use by breastfeeding mothers is considered safe. Nevertheless, each decision to breast-feed should be made after conducting a risk/benefit analysis for each mother and her infant [163].

6.2.2.9 Metformin and Metabolic Syndrome

As explained before, metformin increases insulin sensitivity [89, 100, 103, 166–169] and decreases weight, waist circumference, and BMI [100, 102, 167, 170], particularly if associated with diet and physical exercise.

Some authors state that, without metformin, weight loss (through caloric restriction and increased exercise) is difficult to achieve and maintain [171, 172], due to the weight-preserving and anabolic effects of high insulin [173] and androgens [91].

It was demonstrated that reduction of body weight, BMI, and visceral fat was greater than placebo, and the combination of metformin plus lifestyle intervention was more effective than placebo plus lifestyle intervention [174].

Metformin could act to improve body weight in obese PCOS patients both directly and indirectly:

- Direct effect: on the central nervous system, by modulating appetite in the hypo-thalamus [175]
- Indirect effect: via adipocytokine modification
  Visfatin is the most recently identified adipocytokine, which seems to be prefe-rentially produced by visceral adipose tissue and has insulin-mimetic action [176]. Circulating visfatin levels are higher in patients with PCOS than healthy controls, and it was demonstrated that metformin treatment significantly reduced visfatin levels after 3 months of therapy [177].

It has been suggested that weight loss may be a dose-related response with increased weight loss at higher dose [170]. In fact, comparing two different doses, a significant drop in BMI and waist circumference was seen in those patients using the higher dose [178].

Investigators have reported a greater weight, BMI, and WC reduction in obese patients receiving 2,550 mg/day and concluded that the long-term effect of metfor-min is better with greater dose [170, 179].

Additionally, metformin may slow the progression to type II diabetes melli-tus [66].

This protective effect might be associated with the preservation of pancreatic beta-cell function and appeared to be mediated by a reduction in the secretory demands placed on beta cells by chronic insulin resistance [180].

A recent position statement from the AES (Androgen Excess Society) recom-mended that women with PCOS, regardless of weight, should be screened for IGT or type II diabetes mellitus by an oral glucose tolerance test at their initial presenta-tion and every 2 years thereafter [181].

However, this statement noted that the use of metformin to treat or prevent the progression of IGT could be considered but should not be mandated at this point in time because well-designed RCTs demonstrating efficacy have yet to be conducted

[67]. Moreover, it is important to underline that metformin does not maintain its benefits at a biochemical and clinical level after a 12-month treatment suspension [89].

It is widely known that insulin resistance and consequent metabolic syndrome increase the risk of cardiovascular disease: for this reason, it is very important to consider long-term health when selecting a medical treatment in overweight women with PCOS [182].

PCOS young patients usually do not manifest increased blood pressure values [183], but at menopause women with PCOS have a risk of developing hypertension 2.5-fold higher than age-matched controls [184]: metformin could prevent structural changes that precede hypertension [67]. In fact, it has been shown that metformin improve endothelial function, coronary microvascular function, and coronary flow rate [185].

As explained in previous chapters, dyslipidemia is a typical feature of metabolic syndrome: metformin improves hepatic fatty acid metabolism from lipogenesis toward oxidation.

Different beneficial effects are reported on dyslipidemia in PCOS women [130, 173, 186–192]:

- Decreased total and LDL cholesterol levels
- Decreased triglyceride levels
- Increased HDL cholesterol levels

To prevent vascular consequences, LDL particles should be normalized.

Despite metformin has been shown to improve metabolic alteration, it cannot be considered as first-line therapy [193], but it should be used as an adjunct to lifestyle modification.

Besides ameliorating the metabolic syndrome already present, metformin appears to be also effective in preventing the onset of the metabolic syndrome [194]; a study reported that PCOS women treated with a combination of metformin and controlled diet had significant and sustained improvements in all parameters of the metabolic syndrome over 4 years [195]. Conversely, another study showed that beneficial effects of metformin on the metabolic syndrome, without a specific lifestyle modification regimen, could be sustained over 3 years of routine clinic follow-up [194].

Furthermore, chronic inflammation is one of the PCOS features. Metformin alone reduces circulating levels of CRP (inflammation marker that is usually higher in PCOS women) [196]. It exerts a direct vascular anti-inflammatory effect by dose dependently inhibiting IL-1β-induced release of the pro-inflammatory cytokines IL-6 and IL-8 in endothelial cells, human vascular smooth muscle cells, and macrophages [67, 197].

Endothelial dysfunction, assessed by reduced flow-mediated dilatation, has shown promising results in cardiovascular risk stratification and prognosis [198, 199]. Metformin administration for 6 months in women with PCOS induced a significant increase in flow-mediated dilatation that was restored to normal values [200].

A recent study suggests that metformin decreases serum levels of asymmetric dimethylarginine (ADMA) levels, an endogenous inhibitor of NOS, by concomitant effects on insulin action and androgen levels [201].

Metformin seems to be effective even in decreasing AGE levels, which are oxidative mediators of endothelial dysfunction [134].

Plasminogen activator inhibitor-1 is a pro-thrombotic factor produced by the endothelium that inhibits fibrinolysis and regulates vascular smooth muscle proliferation [202]. Insulin upregulates PAI-1 gene transcription [203] and stimulates hepatic [204] and endothelial PAI-1 production [205]. It has been demonstrated that metformin reduces PAI-1 levels [131–133].

6.2.2.10 Metformin and Hypothyroidism

A recent study stated that in overweight PCOS patients with primary sub-hypothyroidism, treatment with metformin (1,500 mg/day) resulted in a significant fall in TSH and in some cases improvement of hypothyroidism [206].

This is an important finding because hypothyroidism occurs in more than 10 % of PCOS patients [207].

Several mechanisms have been hypothesized:

- A slight increase in the gastrointestinal absorption of levothyroxine (in patients already in treatment with L-thyroxine) [208].
- Influence of changes in body weight, associated with metformin therapy, on TSH levels [209].
- Increase of dopamine in the hypothalamus [210]. Previous studies, in fact, have suggested that there was a disruption of the neuroendocrine mechanisms in women with PCOS, mainly due to a deficiency in hypothalamic dopamine [211].

Further studies are needed to confirm these findings, but some authors suggest starting to treat obese PCOS patients with subclinical hypothyroidism with metformin and to reevaluate their thyroid function after 6 months [206].

6.2.2.11 Metformin Use in Lean PCOS Women

It was revealed that metformin decreases ovarian cytochrome P450c17α activity: this mechanism leads to a reduction of free testosterone serum levels even in lean PCOS women, with a consequent improvement of hyperandrogenism [212].

In fact, it has been demonstrated that women with PCOS who have normal weight or are thin responded to a reduction in insulin release with decreased ovarian androgen production and serum ovarian androgens.

As Nestler highlighted several years ago, metformin treatment of nonobese women leads to [213]:

- Decreased fasting and glucose-stimulated insulin levels
- Decreased basal and GnRH-stimulated LH release
- Decreased ovarian androgen production
- Decreased both serum total and free testosterone concentrations
- Increased serum SHBG concentrations
- Decreased androstenedione and DHEAS levels

Six months of metformin therapy clinically results in beneficial effects in lean PCOS women in terms of resumption of menses, without any remarkable effect on metabolic and cardiovascular risk factors [214].

Moreover, a very recent study suggests that treatment with metformin, for at least 12 weeks prior to, and during, IVF/ICSI, is worth considering as a management approach for nonobese women with PCOS [215].

6.2.2.12 Metformin Use in PCOS Adolescents

Metformin is indicated in patients older than 10 years, 2 years after their menarche.

Few studies demonstrated that metformin improved ovulatory function even in PCOS adolescents [93, 216], as well as hyperandrogenism [217].

As in adult population, metformin is effective in reducing hyperinsulinemia and lipid abnormalities.

A recent study reported that PCOS was the main indication for metformin prescription in UK general practice, even if it is off-label [218].

In the FDA approval process, several studies that demonstrated the safety of metformin use in the adolescent population were conducted.

Contraindications and side effects are the same described for adults.

Even if the literature on metformin in adolescents is limited and the number of studies inconsistent, it is possible that early intervention might prevent the complete spectrum of the syndrome in young overweight girls [219].

However, to date, in adolescent population, the first-step treatment is always the lifestyle modification.

In obese adolescents with PCOS, EP combination pills are the standard of care when lifestyle modification is not effective [220]. EP pills treat hyperandrogenism by increasing SHBG and so decreasing free testosterone; it reduces LH and FSH secretion and decreases ovarian stimulation and androgen production. Progesterone induces menstrual cyclicity and prevents endometrial hyperplasia [221]. However, EP pills do not treat IR or components of the metabolic syndrome [222] and are instead associated with glucose intolerance, decreased insulin sensitivity, abnormal lipid profiles, and CV disease [223, 224].

A recent study compared metformin monotherapy vs. estrogen–progesterone + metformin in the treatment of overweight and obese PCOS adolescents [220]: it was shown that the use of metformin alone was associated with greater decrease in total cholesterol and triglycerides and with a better improvement in weight loss.

These findings suggest that metformin monotherapy is more effective in reducing cardiovascular risk in overweight and obese adolescents with PCOS than the combination with EP pill [220].

6.2.2.13 Metformin + Pioglitazone in PCOS Treatment

Pioglitazone as add-on therapy in metformin-resistant PCOS women (e.g., in women who after 6 months' 1,500–2,500 mg daily metformin treatment fail to improve their metabolic and hyperandrogenemia-related clinical signs) may exert beneficial metabolic (further reduction of IR and glucose levels, improved lipid metabolism, and lowering of carotid intima–media thickness) and antiandrogenic (improved menstrual regularity, significant drop in testosterone and DHEAS levels, increased SHBG, and improved hirsutism score) effects [64, 225, 226].

Moreover, the addition of pioglitazone was not associated with any adverse side effects, such as hepatotoxicity and hypoglycemia [226], providing another valid option for the management of NAFLD and NASH in PCOS women [64].

Pioglitazone safety in women under 18 is not yet established; thus, pioglitazone is not recommended in this female PCOS subgroup. Its safety in pregnancy and lactation is not entirely clear, but it is classified as category C drugs by the FDA due to the fact that studies in animals have shown adverse fetal effects such as IUGR [64].

However, long-term and large-sampled clinical trials are necessary before stating definitive conclusions.

6.2.3 Statins

Statins are competitive inhibitors of HMG-CoA reductase, the rate-limiting enzyme of the cholesterol biosynthesis [227]: inhibition of this enzyme decreases cholesterol synthesis with a compensatory increase in the expression of LDL receptors in the liver. In the general population, statins decrease total cholesterol and LDL cholesterol, and they have antiproliferative and antioxidant features on endothelial cells [228].

Statins reduce plasma triglycerides in a dose-dependent manner, and they also have a modest HDL-raising effect, which is not dose dependent [229, 230].

As dyslipidemia is a component of metabolic syndrome, atorvastatin and simvastatin have been used in PCOS women to investigate their effects on this common syndrome.

To date, there are limited data on the use of statins in PCOS, but short-term use of statins alone or in combination with metformin appears to improve lipid levels in PCOS. In a meta-analysis, statins were more effective than placebo in reducing total cholesterol, LDL, and triglycerides; lipid profile improvement occurred within the first 3 months of treatment, with no further significant change thereafter [231].

A combination of metformin with statins was more successful than metformin alone in lowering fasting glucose, fasting insulin, LDL cholesterol, and triglycerides [232].

Moreover, in the presence of simvastatin, metformin is much more effective in reducing testosterone, DHEAS, hirsutism, and LH and reversing the LH/FSH ratio in patients with PCOS [233].

The mechanisms of action of simvastatin on inhibition of T levels are likely related to the inhibition of the mevalonate pathway [233, 234]. Statins might also decrease the expression of several key enzymes involved in T production: cholesterol side chain cleavage ($P450_{SCC}$), 17α-hydroxylase/17,20-lyase ($P450_{c17}$), and 3β-hydroxysteroid dehydrogenase (3βHSD). Such effects of statins were noted in adrenocortical cells [235, 236]. The mechanisms of these actions might be due to the inhibitory effects of statins on isoprenylation [237], leading to decreased function of small guanosine triphosphatases, such as Ras: statin might abrogate Ras-induced steroidogenesis [236].

Additionally, statins induce inhibition of proliferation of theca interstitial cells and might reduce T output of the ovary by reducing the size of the theca interstitial compartment [233].

Thus, although simvastatin plus metformin could successfully reduce hyperandrogenism, insulin resistance, and lipid profile, its clinical significance is yet to be characterized [233].

However, statins are considered pregnancy category X drugs, and so it is always required to avoid contraception: this represents a very important restriction of use, and it is not a good option of treatment for all PCOS patients who want to get pregnant.

Finally, statins should be reserved only for women with PCOS who have increased LDL cholesterol [238].

6.3   Inositol and Other Supplements

In recent years, more attention has been paid to some supplements, which seem to have an important role in the therapy of PCOS, such as inositol and antioxidant molecules.

6.3.1   Inositol and Its Isomers

Several inositol isomers, and in particular myoinositol (MI) and D-chiro-inositol (DCI), were shown to have insulin-mimetic properties and to be efficient in the treatment of PCOS.

Inositol (cyclohexane-1,2,3,4,5,6-hexol) is a polyol existing under nine stereo-isomeric forms depending on the spatial orientation of its six hydroxyl groups (Fig. 6.1).

Myoinositol is naturally present in animal and plant cells, as free form, as inositol-containing phospholipid (phosphoinositides), or as phytic acid (IP_6) [239].

The greatest amounts of myoinositol in common foods are found in fresh fruits and vegetables and in peas, beans, grains, and nuts [240].

Originally, myoinositol was considered one of the B-complex vitamins, but now it is no more reputed an essential nutrient because it was shown that it is produced in sufficient amount in the human body from D-glucose [241].

It was shown that myoinositol is indispensable for the growth and survival of cells [242] and for the development and function of peripheral nerves [243]; it is essential to bone formation, osteogenesis, and bone mineral density [244], but its therapeutic implications are mainly related to its important role in glucose homeostasis.

A significant part of the ingested myoinositol is consumed in the form of phosphatidylinositol (PI) that may be hydrolyzed by a pancreatic phospholipase A in the intestinal lumen. Ninety-nine percent of the myoinositol ingested is absorbed from the human gastrointestinal tract, through an active transport system involving a Na$^+$/K$^+$-ATPase [239].

Cells mainly derive inositol from three sources:

- De novo biosynthesis from glucose-6-phosphate by 1D-myoinositol-phosphate synthase (MIPS) and inositol monophosphatase (IMPase)
- Dephosphorylation of inositol phosphates derived from breakdown of inositol-containing membrane phospholipids
- Uptake from the extracellular fluid via specialized myoinositol transporters [245]

In vivo, conversion of myoinositol to D-chiro-inositol can occur in tissue expressing the specific epimerase.

Myoinositol and D-chiro-inositol can also be bound components of glycosylphosphatidylinositol (GPI) anchors and of inositol phosphoglycan (IPG) that would constitute second messengers of insulin action in the GPI/IPG pathway [241].

The exact mechanisms of action of MI and DCI with insulin-mimetic activities are still unclear; a presumed mechanism of action implies inositol phosphoglycans (IPGs) containing MI or DCI as insulin mediators [241].

A few studies hypothesized that insulin, other growth factors, and classical hormones stimulated the hydrolysis of glycosylphosphatidylinositol (GPI) generating water-soluble inositol phosphoglycan (IPG) second messenger. The origin of IPG-A is thought to be myoinositol-containing GPI [246].

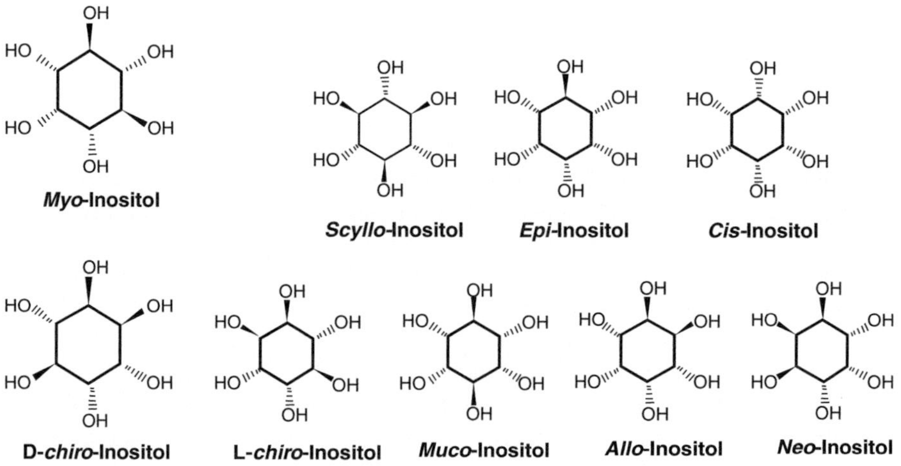

Fig. 6.1 Inositol isomers

One of the most interesting models is the one elaborated by Larner and coworkers in 2010 [247]. According to this model, insulin binding to its receptor (IR) causes the autoactivation of the receptor, and the activated IR can transduce the signal through two parallel signaling pathways, which act together to mediate insulin action in a complementary and synergistic manner [241]:

1. The first one implies the recruitment and activation of substrate of insulin receptor (IRS) by the activated IR. Subsequent protein activations (PI3K, PDK-1) finally lead to PKB-Akt recruitment and activation at the plasma membrane. Activated PKB-Akt induces GLUT-4 translocation to the plasma membrane, improving glucose entry into the cell.
2. When insulin binds to its receptor, the epimerase converts MI molecules to DCI. In the second pathway, the IR is fixed to a G protein itself attached to a phospholipase that catalyzes the hydrolysis of a GPI [248, 249]. The insulin-induced hydrolysis of the GPI releases an inositol phosphoglycan containing D-chiro-inositol (DCI-IPG), which acts as a probable second messenger of insulin (INS-2) mediating insulin effects on glucose oxidative and non-oxidative clearance. INS-2 binds and activates two Mg^{2+}-dependent protein phosphatases: PP2Cα in the cytosol and PDHP in the mitochondria. Activated PP2Cα stimulates glycogen synthase directly and also indirectly through possible activation of PI3K-Akt and subsequent inhibition of GSK3. In the mitochondria, activated PDHP stimulates PDH and so glucose oxidative use [241].

The insulin-sensitizing effect of a MI and DCI supplementation is probably due to their intracellular enhanced availability for the production of membrane IPG precursors; numerous evidences support the hypothesis of a role of inositol glycan insulin second messengers in insulin-mimetic properties of some inositol isomers.

Moreover, it is known that part of MI supplementation effect on insulin sensitivity may come from its partial in vivo intracellular epimerization to DCI [241].

MI intracellular concentration is regulated through processes such as extracellular MI uptake, de novo biosynthesis, regeneration, efflux, and degradation. Alteration of one or several of these processes can lead to inositol intracellular abnormalities [241] in diabetes mellitus: inhibition of cellular MI uptake, altered MI biosynthesis, enhanced MI efflux due to sorbitol intracellular accumulation, and increased MI degradation are putative mechanisms of MI intracellular depletion [250].

Larner et al. noted a decreased urinary excretion of DCI and an increased urinary excretion of MI in humans and monkeys with type II diabetes (ten times higher compared to healthy subjects) [251].

The ratio of MI/DCI is regulated by an epimerase that converts MI into DCI [252], and Larner showed that each organ has a specific MI/DCI ratio [253].

Altered ratios of increased myoinositol to decreased D-chiro-inositol in urine have even been proposed as an index of insulin resistance in humans [254]: a deficit in MI to DCI epimerization activity, due to an epimerase-type enzyme, was supposed [249, 255].

Excessive urinary MI excretion could reduce MI plasma level and subsequently emphasize MI intracellular depletion, particularly in tissues heavily dependent on extracellular MI import [241]. Decreased production of DCI from MI reduces the availability of intracellular DCI for its incorporation into IPGs (particularly, DCI-IPG), probable downstream second messengers of insulin.

Furthermore, the decreased DCI content in insulin target tissues could reduce insulin signal transduction involving IPGs, in order to contribute to insulin resistance in those tissues. Depleted plasma levels of DCI observed in PCOS patients underline the correlation between impaired plasma DCI and insulin resistance [241].

Thus, insulin resistance is associated with:

1. Abnormally low levels of DCI in urine, plasma, and insulin target tissues (liver, muscle, fat)
2. Excessive MI urinary excretion
3. Intracellular MI deficiency in insulin-sensitive tissues (Fig. 6.2)

On the contrary, more recently (in 2006) Nestler proposed that, in a woman with PCOS, an initial genetic or environmental insult causing insulin resistance leads to a compensatory hyperinsulinemia. The latter induces a defect that increases renal clearance of DCI, and this leads to a reduction in circulating DCI and its availability to tissue. The consequence is an intracellular deficiency of DCI and of DCI-IPG, a mediator of insulin action.

Diminished release of DCI-IPG in response to stimulation by insulin results in a further decrease in insulin sensitivity [256] (Fig. 6.3).

In 2010, Baillargeon et al. [257] showed that when plasma glucose is maintained at stable levels and plasma insulin is acutely raised and maintained at constant levels, the circulating DCI-IPG insulin mediator is released rapidly and briefly in normal women. Conversely, this coupling between insulin action and DCI-IPG release was entirely absent in obese women with PCOS: the release of bioactive DCI-IPG was significantly lower in obese PCOS women [257].

Possible explanations for these findings are a deficit in intracellular DCI or DCI-IPG and/or a defect in incorporation of the substrate DCI with membrane phosphoglycans to generate DCI-IPG mediator [257].

The possibility that a deficit in circulating DCI, or its precursor MI, is responsible for defective insulin-stimulated release of DCI-IPG mediator in PCOS is supported by the findings that oral supplementation with DCI [258–260] or MI [261, 262] to both lean and obese PCOS women improved their insulin resistance and clinical symptoms.

Moreover, defective DCI-IPG release in response to insulin could be due to a qualitative (rather than quantitative) defect in the insulin signaling mechanism that activates DCI-IPG mediator release from the membrane: there may be a primary defect in the union of the insulin receptor β-unit to the G protein or a defect in G-protein activation of phospholipase C [257].

This observation fits with Cheang et al. data [263]: they showed, in a number of hyperinsulinemic PCOS patients who did not respond to DCI treatment, the absence

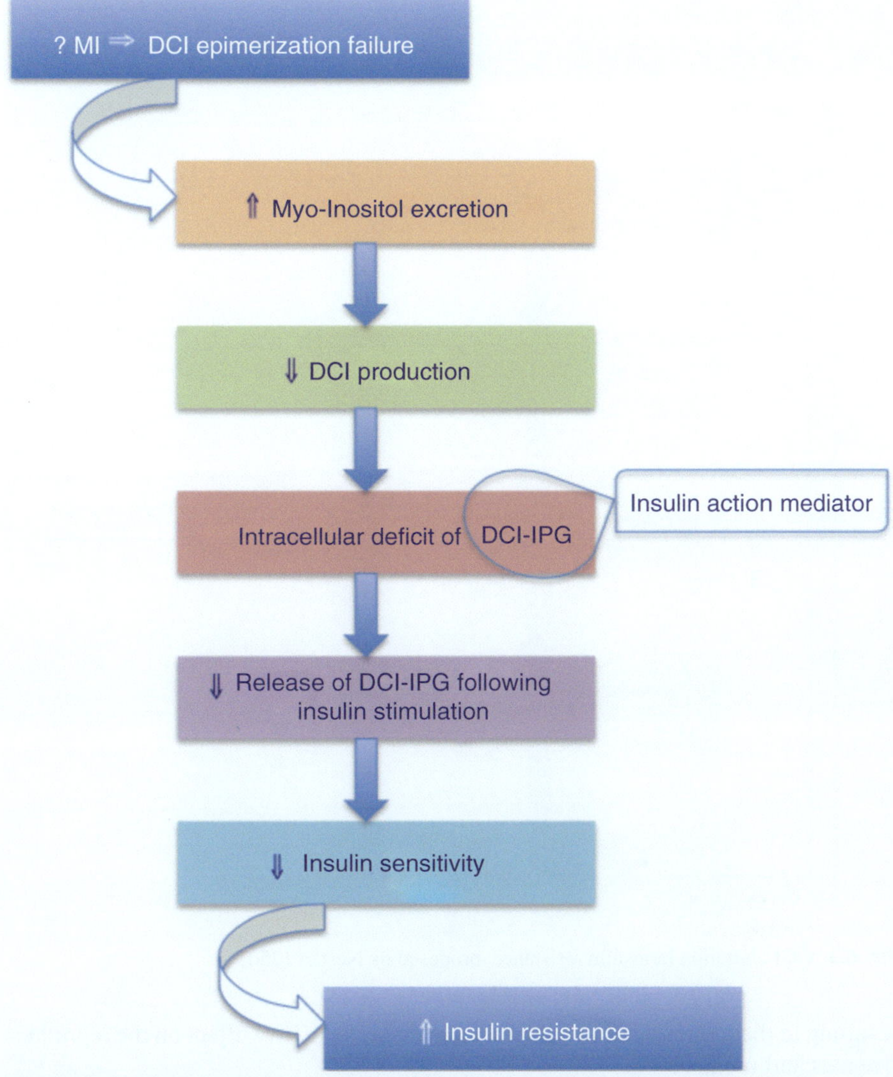

Fig. 6.2 MI and DCI alteration in insulin resistance, proposed by Larner [251]

of changes in DCI-IPG release suggesting that a functional defect rather than a simple inositol nutritional deficiency might be present [263, 264].

6.3.1.1 Inositol as Treatment for PCOS

A supplementation with myoinositol or D-chiro-inositol was found to be safe and effective in improving metabolic and hormonal parameters in PCOS patients: the main mechanism of action is based on improving insulin sensitivity of target tissues,

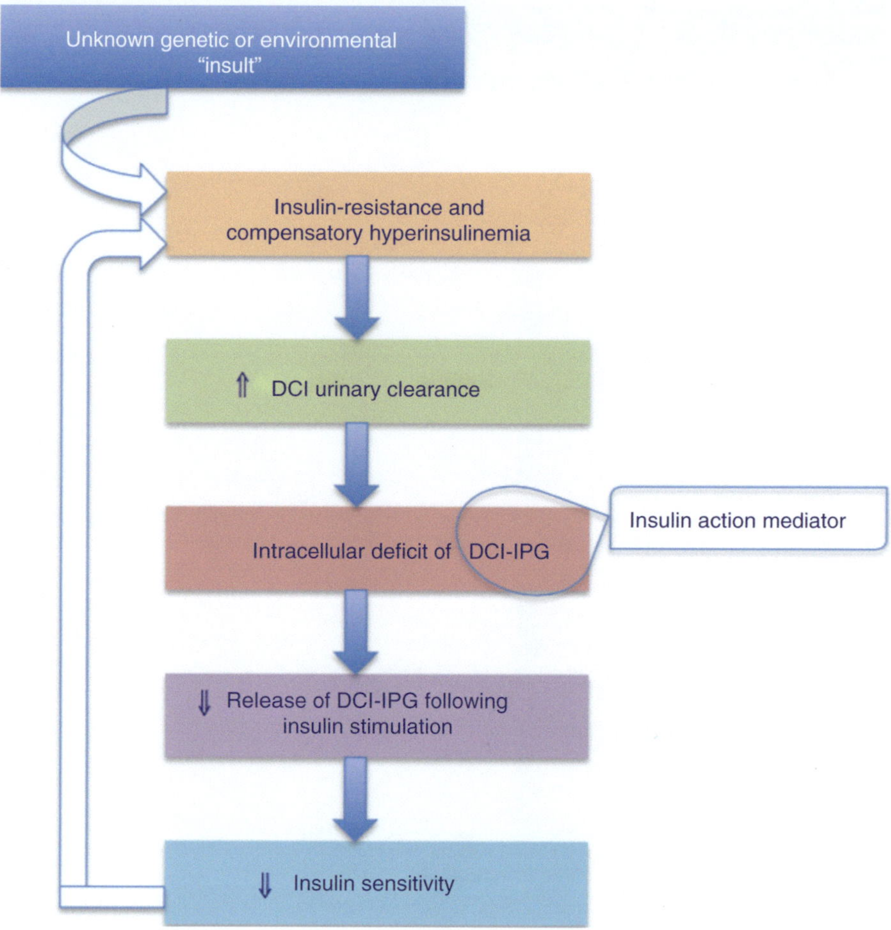

Fig. 6.3 DCI alteration in insulin resistance, proposed by Nestler [256]

resulting in the reduction of insulinemia which has a positive effect on the reproductive axis and metabolism.

One of the first studies was conducted in 1999 by Nestler et al. [258], who found that the administration of D-chiro-inositol to women with polycystic ovary syndrome decreased the insulin response to orally administered glucose; simultaneously with the reduction in insulin secretion, women who received DCI had a significant improvement in ovulatory function and decreased serum androgen concentrations [258].

It was demonstrated in various studies that both DCI and MI are able to:

- Reduce LH levels, LH/FSH ratio, and testosterone levels [258, 265–268].
- Restore spontaneous ovulation and menstrual cycles [258, 260, 262, 265, 269].
- Improve cutaneous disorders of hyperandrogenism, reducing hirsutism and acne score [266].

- Decrease HOMA index [264, 265, 267].
- Reduce systolic arterial blood pressure [267, 268].
- Reduce leptin, LDL cholesterol levels, and triglycerides [269].
- Increase HDL cholesterol level [260, 269].

In view of all these findings, recently we conducted a research to evaluate the clinical, endocrine, and metabolic response of young women with PCOS, treated for 12 weeks with DCI.

From a clinical point of view, our study has highlighted a significant retrieval of menstrual cycle regularity ($p < 0.001$) in a rate higher than 60 % in patients treated and a significant improvement of acne score ($p < 0.05$) in patients with D-chiro-inositol treatment. Moreover, there was a significant decrease of triglyceride ($p < 0.05$) and basal insulin serum levels ($p < 0.05$) in patients treated with D-chiro-inositol [270].

Another clinical study of our group has shown that the administration of D-chiro-inositol in association with estro-progestins (0.03 mg of ethinyl estradiol and 3 mg of drospirenone) leads to a significant decrease of acne already from the second month of treatment, amplifying earlier the effects of oral contraceptives [271].

In literature no side effects after MI or DCI administration were reported when clinical dosage was used (max 1 g of DCI or 4 g of MI). Clinical trial data indicate that adverse events related to inositol treatment are gastrointestinal symptoms (nausea, flatus, loose stools, diarrhea) at a dose of 12 g/day or higher [272].

Moreover, MI or DCI supplementation was demonstrated to be effective in reducing the risk of gestational diabetes (GB) in PCOS women [273, 274], even if more studies are needed to confirm these preliminary data.

Finally, we suggest the use of MI (4 g die) or DCI (1 g die) as first-line treatment for those lean PCOS patients suffering from oligomenorrhea and mild hyperandrogenism. Combined therapy with diet, exercise, and metformin is reserved for insulin-resistant and overweight PCOS patients with oligomenorrhea and moderate hyperandrogenism.

6.3.1.2 Inositol and Oocyte Quality

Myoinositol function is also linked to the important role of IP3 in oocyte development and maturation [275, 276].

Oocyte cycle is usually arrested at metaphase of the second meiotic division. Calcium release mechanisms are shown to undergo modification during oogenesis, and maximal sensitivity of calcium release is acquired during the final stages of oocyte maturation: after fertilization, an increased level of intracellular Ca^{++} occurs, and subsequent conclusion of meiosis [277, 278].

It was experimentally observed that immature oocytes (germinal vesicles or oocytes undergone in vitro process of maturation) contain a number of IP3 receptors less than those matured in vivo, leading to a reduction in Ca^{++} intracytoplasmic rise.

The disposal of Ca^{++} from intracellular deposits is required for the oocyte's activation that is manifested by the exocytosis of cortical granules, the perpetuation of the second meiotic division, the extrusion of the II polar body, the formation of two pronuclei, and the activation of protein synthesis from maternal RNA to prime the first mitosis.

Inositol depletion dramatically reduces transduction signal mechanisms mediated by IP3, altering the dynamics linked to the intracellular Ca^{++} fluctuations.

Myoinositol supplementation may prevent this block and promote meiotic progression of the germinal vesicles; in fact, it was demonstrated that follicles containing high levels of MY, dosed in follicular fluid, present oocytes of good quality, and this may be related to a close correspondence between MI and inositol phosphates, necessary during oocyte maturation PIP2-mediated [279].

In human follicular fluid a greater concentration of myoinositol is a marker of good oocyte quality.

A recent clinical trial showed that only MI rather than DCI is able to improve oocyte quality [280]; the reason was explained by the "DCI paradox in the ovary" [281]: it is explained that "ovaries in PCOS patients likely present an enhanced MI to DCI epimerization that leads to a MI tissue depletion; this, in turn, could eventually be responsible for the poor oocyte quality characteristic of these patients" [282].

However, this hypothesis has yet to be confirmed: in fact, even DCI supplementation has shown a significant improvement in oocyte quality.

One of our recent studies showed that, in patients with PCOS, treatment with myoinositol and folic acid, compared to only acid folic treatment, reduces the number of germinal vesicles and degenerated oocytes at the time of oocytes' pickup, without affecting the total number of oocytes retrieved. Moreover, an increased number of transferred embryos of good quality and a reduced amount of FSHR IU administered for the ovulation induction were shown [283].

These results were consistent with those found in other studies [284], suggesting the positive effect that myoinositol plays in the development of mature oocytes.

Furthermore, recent data demonstrate that by providing both MI and DCI in a physiological ratio (40:1), hormonal and metabolic imbalances are treated much more quickly compared to MI alone [252], especially in overweight PCOS patients who need to control insulin levels and increase ovarian MI content, reducing the risk of developing a metabolic disease [285, 286].

6.3.2　Antioxidants

Polycystic ovary syndrome is also associated with decreased antioxidant concentrations, and it is considered an oxidative state [287].

The decrease in mitochondrial O_2 consumption and GSH levels along with increased ROS production explains the mitochondrial dysfunction in PCOS patients [288]. The mononuclear cells of women with PCOS are increased in this inflammatory state [289], which occurs mostly in response to hyperglycemia and C-reactive protein (CRP) [290].

Physiological hyperglycemia generates increased levels of ROS from mononuclear cells, which activate the release of TNF-α and increase inflammatory transcription factor NF-kappa B. As a result, concentrations of TNF-α, a known mediator of insulin resistance, are further increased [290].

Oxidative stress and inflammation promotes hyperandrogenism, which augments the inflammatory load [289].

Oxidative stress promotes its effects causing damage to follicular proteins by the marking of free thiol groups [291].

Furthermore, reactive oxygen species (ROS) has been considered to play a critical role in the success of different IVF techniques. ROS are produced within the follicle, especially during the ovulatory process [292], and it is believed that oxidative stress may be a cause of poor oocyte quality [293]. In fact, high levels of oxidants, as H_2O_2, have been found in fragmented embryos [294].

MI and DCI are considered an effective therapy for PCOS women even for its antioxidant activity.

A recent study demonstrated that MI treatment positively affected the oxidative status of red blood cells (RBC), as shown by the partial restoration of GSH contents and the reduction of both band 3 Tyr-P levels and protein glutathionylation [295].

Moreover, there is evidence that melatonin plays an important role in the regulation of reproductive activity [296], and high levels of melatonin have been found in human preovulatory follicular fluid in concentrations that are almost threefold higher than serum levels [297–299]. It is known that melatonin and its metabolites are potent direct free radical scavengers [300–303] and indirect antioxidants, due to their ability to modulate gene transcription for antioxidant enzymes [304].

An Italian study demonstrated that, in patients undergoing IVF, treatment with melatonin plus myoinositol and folic acid reduced the number of germinal vesicles and degenerated oocytes and increased the number of top-quality embryos, compared to the therapy with only MI [305].

Other two important antioxidant molecules are SOD (superoxide dismutase) and ALA (α-lipoic acid).

Therapeutic strategy to reduce the oxidative stress includes diet rich in vegetables, weight reduction, physical exercise, smoking cessation, alcohol consumption reduction, and adequate number of sleeping hours.

6.3.3   Vitamin D

Vitamin D has pleiotropic effects on a large spectrum of intracellular regulatory processes, including insulin metabolism, or intrinsic apoptotic pathway, on both classical and nonclassical tissues, such as the ovary [306].

Moreover, as explained previously, calcium has an important role in follicle development, and both calcium and vitamin D deficiencies are considered as potential risk factors for insulin resistance and obesity [307–310].

Hypovitaminosis D was found in about 80 % of PCOS women [311, 312].

Supplementation of vitamin D (50,000 IU/week) and calcium (1 g/day) seems to support the positive effect of metformin therapy, with greater results in restoring normal menstrual regularity and improving hyperandrogenism symptoms, weight loss, and follicle maturation compared to metformin treatment alone [311].

Further studies are needed to confirm these data in order to use vitamin D + calcium supplementation as routine PCOS treatment protocol.

6.3.4   Glucomannan

Recently, glucomannan has been introduced as supplement for insulin resistance treatment.

Glucomannan is a high-molecular-weight polysaccharide obtained from tubers of *Amorphophallus konjac*: it consists of molecules of D-glucose and D-mannose, and it is soluble and absorbs water up to 200 times its weight.

Glucomannan exerts its activity by increasing the viscosity of food bolus during digestion: it creates a viscous gel that makes the bolus smooth and soft, and it forms a nondigestible coating around food particles.

This leads to a decreased time of food permanence inside the gastrointestinal tract: as main consequence, the action of digestive enzymes is partially avoided, resulting in reduced absorption of nutrients [313, 314].

Thus, glucomannan slows both lipid and carbohydrate absorption, reducing total and LDL cholesterol [315].

In diabetic patients, it is able to reduce postprandial glycemia and insulinemia [316].

Moreover, glucomannan increases the secretion of glucagon-like peptide 1 (GLP1), cholecystokinin (CCK), and peptide YY (PYY) [317], induces satiation and satiety [318], and preserves weight loss [319].

Minor adverse effects are normally GI related and include diarrhea, flatulence, and bloating.

Recently, an Italian study has shown that the association inositol–glucomannan may represent a good therapeutic strategy in the treatment of PCOS women with insulin resistance [320].

References

1. O'Connor A, Gibney J, Roche HM (2010) Metabolic and hormonal aspects of polycystic ovary syndrome: the impact of diet. Proc Nutr Soc 69:628–635
2. Stansbury J (2012) The PCOS health & nutrition guide: includes 125 recipes for managing polycystic ovarian syndrome. Robert Rose, ISBN: 9780778804055
3. Andersen P, Seljeflot I, Abdelnoor M et al (1995) Increased insulin sensitivity and fibrinolytic capacity after dietary intervention in obese women with polycystic ovary syndrome. Metabolism 44:611–616
4. Moran LJ, Noakes M, Clifton PM et al (2003) Dietary composition in restoring reproductive and metabolic physiology in overweight women with polycystic ovary syndrome. J Clin Endocrinol Metab 88:812–819
5. Crosignani PG, Colombo M, Vegetti W et al (2003) Overweight and obese anovulatory patients with polycystic ovaries: parallel improvements in anthropometric indices, ovarian physiology and fertility rate induced by diet. Hum Reprod 18:1928–1932

6. Herriot AM, Whitcroft S, Jeanes Y (2008) A retrospective audit of patients with polycystic ovary syndrome: the effects of a reduced glycaemic load diet. J Hum Nutr Diet 21(4):337–345
7. Marsh K, Brand-Miller J (2005) The optimal diet for women with polycystic ovary syndrome? Br J Nutr 94:154–165
8. Farshchi H, Rane A, Love A, Kennedy RL (2007) Diet and nutrition in polycystic ovary syndrome (PCOS): pointers for nutritional management. J Obstet Gynaecol 27:762–773
9. Liepa GU, Sengupta A, Karsies D (2008) Polycystic ovary syndrome (PCOS) and other androgen excess-related conditions: can changes in dietary intake make a difference? Nutr Clin Pract 23:63–71
10. Diamanti-Kandarakis E, Katsikist I, Piperi C et al (2007) Effect of long-term orlistat treatment on serum levels of advanced glycation end-products in women with polycystic ovary syndrome. Clin Endocrinol (Oxf) 66:103–109
11. Elsenbruch S, Benson S, Hahn S et al (2006) Determinants of emotional distress in women with polycystic ovary syndrome. Hum Reprod 21:1092–1099
12. Jayagopal V, Kilpatrick ES et al (2005) Orlistat is as beneficial as metformin in the treatment of polycystic ovarian syndrome. J Clin Endocrinol Metabol 90:729–733
13. Gower BA, Chandler-Laney P, Ovalle F et al (2013) Favourable metabolic effects of a eucaloric lower-carbohydrate diet in women with PCOS. Clin Endocrinol (Oxf) 79(4):550–557
14. Sharman MJ, Gomez AL, Kraemer WJ, Volek JS (2004) Very low-carbohydrate and low-fat diets affect fasting lipids and post-prandial lipemia differently in overweight men. J Nutr 134:880–885
15. McAuley KA, Hopkins CM, Smith KJ et al (2005) Comparison of high-fat and high-protein diets with a high-carbohydrate diet in insulin-resistant obese women. Diabetologia 48:8–16
16. Parker B, Noakes M, Luscombe N, Clifton P (2002) Effect of a high-protein, high-monounsaturated fat weight loss diet on glycemic control and lipid levels in type 2 diabetes. Diabetes Care 25:425–430
17. Kwiterovich PO, Vining EPG et al (2003) Effect of a high-fat ketogenic diet on plasma levels of lipids, lipoproteins, and apolipoproteins in children. JAMA 290:912–920
18. Jarvi AE, Karlstrom BE, Granfeldt YE et al (1999) Improved glycemic control and lipid profile and normalized fibrinolytic activity on a low-glycemic index diet in type 2 diabetic patients. Diabetes Care 22:10–18
19. Jenkins DJ, Wolever TM et al (1985) Low glycemic index carbohydrate foods in the management of hyperlipidemia. Am J Clin Nutr 42:604–617
20. Liu S, Willett WC, Stampfer MJ et al (2000) A prospective study of dietary glycemic load, carbohydrate intake and risk of coronary heart disease in US women. Am J Clin Nutr 71:1455–1461
21. Salmeron J, Manson JE, Stampfer MJ et al (1997) Dietary fibre, glycemic load, and risk of non-insulin-dependent diabetes mellitus in women. J Am Med Assoc 277:472–477
22. Brynes AE, Edwards MC, Ghatei MA et al (2003) A randomized four-intervention crossover study investigating the effect of carbohydrates on daytime profiles of insulin, glucose, non-esterified fatty acids and triacylglycerols in middle-aged men. Br J Nutr 89:207–218
23. Marsh KA, Steinbeck KS, Atkinson FS et al (2010) Effect of a low glycemic index compared with a conventional healthy diet on polycystic ovary syndrome. Am J Clin Nutr 92:83–92
24. Jenkins D, Wolever T, Bacon S (1980) Diabetic diets: high carbohydrate combined with high fiber. Am J Clin Nutr 33(8):1729–1733
25. Simpson HC, Simpson RW, Lousley S et al (1981) A high carbohydrate leguminous fiber diet improves all aspects of diabetic control. Lancet 1(8210):1–5
26. Leidy HJ, Bossingham MJ, Mattes RD, Campbell W (2009) Increased dietary protein consumed at breakfast leads to an initial and sustained feeling of fullness during energy restriction compared to other meal times. Br J Nutr 101:798–803
27. Veldhorst M, Smeets A et al (2008) Protein-induced satiety: effects and mechanisms of different proteins. Physiol Behav 94:300–307
28. Leidy HJ, Racki EM (2010) The addition of a protein-rich breakfast and its effects on acute appetite control and food intake in "breakfast-skipping" adolescent. Int J Obes 34:1125–1133

29. Stern L, Iqbal N et al (2004) The effects of low-carbohydrate versus conventional weight loss diets in severely obese adults: one-year follow-up of a randomized trial. Ann Intern Med 140:778–785
30. Kasim-Karakas S, Almario RU, Gregory L et al (2004) Metabolic and endocrine effects of a polyunsaturated fatty acid-rich diet in polycystic ovary syndrome. J Clin Endocrinol Metab 89(2):615–620
31. Kerver JM, Yang EJ, Obayashi S et al (2006) Meal and snack patterns are associated with dietary intake of energy and nutrients in US adults. J Am Diet Assoc 106:46–53
32. Farshchi H, Taylor M, Macdonald I (2004) Regular meal frequency creates more appropriate insulin sensitivity and lipid profiles compared with irregular meal frequency in healthy lean women. Eur J Clin Nutr 58:1071–1077
33. Farshchi H, Taylor M, Macdonald I (2005) Deleterious effects of omitting breakfast on insulin sensitivity and fasting lipid profiles in healthy lean women. Am J Clin Nutr 81:388–396
34. Panidis D, Tziomalos K et al (2013) Lifestyle intervention and anti-obesity therapies in the polycystic ovary syndrome: impact on metabolism and fertility. Endocrine 44:583–590
35. Jakubowics D, Barnea M, Wainstein J, Froy O (2013) Effects of caloric intake timing on insulin resistance and hyperandrogenism in lean women with polycystic ovary syndrome. Clin Sci 125:423–432
36. Jenkins DJ, Wolever TM, Taylor RH et al (1981) Glycemic index of foods: a physiological basis for carbohydrate exchange. Am J Clin Nutr 34(3):362–366
37. Jenkins DJ, Kendall CW, McKeown-Eyssen G et al (2008) Effect of a low-glycemic index or a high-cereal fiber diet on type 2 diabetes: a randomized trial. JAMA 300(23):2742–2753
38. Brouns F, Bjorck I, Frayn KN et al (2005) Glycaemic index methodology. Nutr Res Rev 18(1):145–171
39. Glycemic load defined. Glycemic Research Institute. Retrieved 8 Feb 2013
40. Holt S, Brand-Miller JC, Petocz P (1997) An insulin index of foods: the insulin demand generated by 1000-kJ portions of common foods. Am J Clin Nutr 66(5):1264–1276
41. Palomba S, Giallauria F, Falbo A et al (2008) Structured exercise training programme versus hypocaloric hyperproteic diet in obese polycystic ovary syndrome patients with anovulatory infertility: a 24 week pilot study. Hum Reprod 23:642–650
42. Hawley JA (2004) Exercise as a therapeutic intervention for the prevention and treatment of insulin resistance. Diabetes Metab Res Rev 20:383–393
43. Farrell K, Antoni MH (2010) Insulin resistance, obesity, inflammation, and depression in polycystic ovary syndrome: biobehavioral mechanisms and interventions. Fertil Steril 94:1565–1574
44. Giallauria F, Palomba L, Maresca L et al (2008) Exercise training improves autonomic function and inflammatory pattern in women with polycystic ovary syndrome (PCOS). Clin Endocrinol (Oxf) 69:792–798
45. Thomson RL, Buckley JD, Noakes M et al (2008) The effect of a hypocaloric diet with and without exercise training on body composition, cardiometabolic risk profile, and reproductive function in overweight and obese women with polycystic ovary syndrome. J Clin Endocrinol Metab 93:3373–3380
46. Moran LJ, Pasquali R, Teede HJ et al (2009) Treatment of obesity in polycystic ovary syndrome: a position statement of the Androgen Excess and Polycystic Ovary Syndrome Society. Fertil Steril 92:1966–1982
47. Practice Committee of the American Society for Reproductive Medicine. Use of insulin sensitizing agents in the treatment of polycystic ovary syndrome. Fertil Steril 2008;90:S69–S73
48. Wild RA, Carmina E, Diamanti-Kandarakis E et al (2010) Assessment of cardiovascular risk and prevention of cardiovascular disease in women with the polycystic ovary syndrome: a consensus statement by the Androgen Excess and Polycystic Ovary Syndrome (AE-PCOS) Society. J Clin Endocrinol Metab 95:2038–2049
49. Antonucci T, Whitcomb R, McLain R et al (1998) Impaired glucose tolerance is normalized by treatment with the thiazolidinedione troglitazone. Diabetes Care 20:188–193

50. Lehmann JM, Moore LB, Smith-Oliver TA et al (1995) An antidiabetic thiazolidinedione is a high affinity ligand for peroxisome proliferator activated receptor gamma (PPAR gamma). J Biol Chem 270:12953–12956
51. Yki-Jarvinen H (2004) Thiazolidinediones. N Engl J Med 351:1106–1118
52. Ehrmann D, Schneider DJ, Sobel BE (1997) Troglitazone improves defects in insulin action, insulin secretion, ovarian steroidogenesis and fibrinolysis in women with polycystic ovary syndrome. J Clin Endocrinol Metab 82:2108–2116
53. Dunaif A, Scott D, Finegood D et al (1996) The insulin sensitizing agent troglitazone improves metabolic and reproductive abnormalities in the polycystic ovary syndrome. J Clin Endocrinol Metab 81:3299–3306
54. Azziz R, Ehrmann D, Legro RS et al (2001) Troglitazone improves ovulation and hirsutism in the polycystic ovary syndrome: a multicenter, double blind, placebo-controlled trial. J Clin Endocrinol Metab 86:1626–1632
55. Belli SH, Graffigna MN, Oneto A et al (2004) Effects of rosiglitazone on insulin resistance, growth factors, and reproductive disturbances in women with polycystic ovary syndrome. Fertil Steril 81:624–629
56. Brettenthaler N, De Geyter C, Huber PR, Keller U (2004) Effect of the insulin sensitizer pioglitazone on insulin resistance, hyperandrogenism, and ovulatory dysfunction in women with polycystic ovary syndrome. J Clin Endocrinol Metab 89:3835–3840
57. Grover A, Yalamas MA (2011) Metformin or thiazolidinedione therapy in PCOS? Nat Rev Endocrinol 7:128–129
58. Aroda RV, Ciaraldi TP, Burke P et al (2008) Metabolic and hormonal changes induced by pioglitazone in polycystic ovary syndrome: a randomized, placebo-controlled clinical trial. J Clin Endocrinol Metab 94:469–476
59. Mather KJ, Funahashi T, Matsuzawa Y et al (2008) Diabetes prevention program adiponectin, and progression to diabetes in the diabetes prevention program. Diabetes 57:980–986
60. Glintborg D, Hojlund K, Anderson M et al (2008) Soluble DC36 and risk markers of insulin resistance and atherosclerosis are elevated in polycystic ovary syndrome and significantly reduced during pioglitazone treatment. Diabetes Care 31:328–334
61. Romualdi D, Guido M, Ciampelli M et al (2003) Selective effects of pioglitazone on insulin and androgen abnormalities in normo- and hyperinsulinaemic obese patients with polycystic ovary syndrome. Hum Reprod 18:1210–1218
62. Asadipooya K, Kalantar-Hormozi M, Nabipour I (2012) Pioglitazone reduces central obesity in polycystic ovary syndrome women. Gynecol Endocrinol 28:16–19
63. Glintborg D, Hermann AP, Andersen M et al (2006) Effect of pioglitazone on glucose metabolism and luteinizing hormone secretion in women with polycystic ovary syndrome. Fertil Steril 86:385–397
64. Valsamakis G, Lois K, Kumar S, Mastorakos G (2013) Metabolic and other effects of pioglitazone as an add-on therapy to metformin in the treatment of polycystic ovary syndrome (PCOS). Hormones 12(3):363–378
65. Sepilian V, Negamani M (2005) Effects of rosiglitazone in obese women with polycystic ovary syndrome and severe insulin resistance. J Clin Endocrinol Metab 90:60–65
66. Nestler JE (2008) Metformin for the treatment of the polycystic ovary syndrome. N Engl J Med 358:47–54
67. Palomba S, Falbo A, Zullo F, Orio F (2009) Evidence-based and potential benefits of metformin in the polycystic ovary syndrome: a comprehensive review. Endocr Rev 30(1):1–50
68. Jamieson MA (2002) Opinions in pediatric and adolescent gynecology. J Pediatr Adolesc Gynecol 15:109–114
69. Bailey C, Turner R (1996) Metformin. N Engl J Med 334:574–579
70. Morin-Papunen LC, Koivunen RM, Ruokonen A, Martikainen HK (1998) Metformin therapy improves the menstrual pattern with minimal endocrine and metabolic effects in women with polycystic ovary syndrome. Fertil Steril 69:691–696

71. Musi N, Hirshmen MF, Nygren J et al (2002) Metformin increases AMP activated protein kinase activity in skeletal muscle of subjects with type 2 diabetes. Diabetes 51:2074–2081

72. Zhou G, Myers R, Li Y et al (2001) Role of AMP activated protein kinase in mechanism of metformin action. J Clin Invest 108:1167–1174

73. Zou MH, Kirkpatrick SS, Davis BJ et al (2004) Activation of the AMP activated protein kinase by the anti-diabetic drug metformin in vivo. J Biol Chem 279:43940–43951

74. Elisa E, Sander V, Lucchetti CG et al (2006) The mechanisms involved in the action of metformin in regulating ovarian function in hyperandrogenized mice. Mol Hum Reprod 12:475–481

75. Cibula D, Fanta M, Vrbikova J et al (2005) The effect of combination therapy with metformin and combined oral contraceptives (COC) versus COC alone on insulin sensitivity, hyperandrogenemia, SHBG and lipids in PCOS patients. Hum Reprod 20:180–184

76. Mathur R, Alexander CJ, Yano J et al (2008) Use of metformin in polycystic ovary syndrome. Am J Obstet Gynecol 199(6):596–609

77. Genazzani AD, Strucchi C, Luis M et al (2006) Metformin administration modulates neurosteroids secretion in non-obese amenorrhoic patients with polycystic ovary syndrome. Gynecol Endocrinol 22:36–43

78. Attia GR, Rainey WE, Carr BR (2001) Metformin directly inhibits androgen production in human thecal cells. Fertil Steril 76:517–524

79. Erickson GF, Magoffin DA, Cragun JR, Chang RJ (1990) The effects of insulin and insulin-like growth factors-I and – II on estradiol production by granulosa cells of polycystic ovaries. J Clin Endocrinol Metab 70:894–902

80. Catteau-Jonard S, Jasmin SP, Leclerc A et al (2008) Anti-Mullerian hormone, its receptor, FSH receptor, and androgen receptor genes are overexpressed by granulosa cells from stimulated follicles in women with polycystic ovary syndrome. J Clin Endocrinol Metab 93(11):4456–4461

81. Gonzalez-Fernandez R, Pena O, Hernandez J et al (2011) Patients with endometriosis and patients with poor ovarian reserve have abnormal follicle-stimulating hormone receptor signaling pathways. Fertil Steril 95(7):2373–2378

82. Rice S, Elia A, Jawad Z et al (2013) Metformin inhibits follicle-stimulating hormone (FSH) action in human granulosa cells: relevance to polycystic ovary syndrome. J Clin Endocrinol Metab 98(9):E1491–E1500

83. Dunn CJ, Peters DH (1995) Metformin. A review of its pharmacological properties and therapeutic use in non-insulin-dependent diabetes mellitus. Drugs 49:721–749

84. Palomba S, Falbo A, Orio F et al (2008) Efficacy predictors for metformin and clomiphene citrate treatment in anovulatory infertile patients with polycystic ovary syndrome. Fertil Steril. doi:10.1016/j.fertnstert.2008.03.011

85. Maciel GAR, Soares Junior JM, Alves L, da Motta E et al (2004) Non obese women with polycystic ovary syndrome respond better than obese women to treatment with metformin. Fertil Steril 81(2):355–360

86. Poretsky L, Cataldo NA, Rosenwaks Z, Giudice LC (1999) The insulin-related ovarian regulatory system in health and disease. Endocr Rev 20:535–582

87. Aubuchon M, Kunselman AR, Schlaff WD et al (2011) Metformin and/or clomiphene do not adversely affect liver or renal function in women with polycystic ovary syndrome. J Clin Endocrinol Metab 96(10):E1645–E1649

88. Preiss D, Sattar N, Harborne L et al (2008) The effects of 8 months of metformin on circulating GGT and ALT levels in obese women with polycystic ovarian syndrome. Int J Clin Pract 62:1337–1343

89. Palomba S, Falbo A, Russo T et al (2007) Insulin sensitivity after metformin suspension in normal-weight women with polycystic ovary syndrome. J Clin Endocrinol Metab 92:3128–3135

90. Aruna J, Mittal S, Kumar S et al (2004) Metformin therapy in women with polycystic ovary syndrome. Int J Gynecol Obstet 87:237–241

91. Glueck CJ, Wang P, Fontaine R et al (2001) Metformin to restore normal menses in oligo-amenorrheic teenage girls with polycystic ovary syndrome (PCOS). J Adolesc Health 29:160–169
92. Velazquez EM, Mendoza S, Harmer T et al (1994) Metformin therapy in polycystic ovary syndrome reduces hyperinsulinemia, insulin resistance, hyperandrogenemia, and systolic blood pressure, while facilitating normal menses and pregnancy. Metabolism 43(5):647–654
93. Moghetti P, Castello R, Negri C et al (2000) Metformin effects on clinical features, endocrine and metabolic profiles, and insulin sensitivity in polycystic ovary syndrome: a randomized, double-blind, placebo-controlled 6-month trial, followed by open, long-term clinical evaluation. J Clin Endocrinol Metab 85:139–146
94. Giudice LC (2006) Endometrium in PCOS: implantation and predisposition to endocrine CA. Best Pract Res Clin Endocrinol Metab 20:235–244
95. Palomba S, Russo T, Orio F Jr et al (2006) Uterine effects of metformin administration in anovulatory women with polycystic ovary syndrome. Hum Reprod 21:457–465
96. Palomba S, Russo T, Orio F Jr et al (2006) Uterine effects of clomiphene citrate in women with polycystic ovary syndrome: a prospective controlled study. Hum Reprod 21:2823–2829
97. Ajossa S, Guerriero S, Paoletti AM et al (2002) The antiandrogenic effect of flutamide improves uterine perfusion in women with polycystic ovary syndrome. Fertil Steril 77:1136–1140
98. Lupulescu A (1993) Estrogen use and cancer risk: a review. Exp Clin Endocrinol 101:204–214
99. Pavelic J, Radakovic B, Pavelic K (2007) Insulin-like growth factor 2 and its receptors (IGF 1R and IGF 2R/mannose 6-phosphate) in endometrial adenocarcinoma. Gynecol Oncol 105:727–735
100. Tan S, Hahn S, Benson S et al (2007) Metformin improves polycystic ovary syndrome symptoms irrespective of pre-treatment insulin resistance. Eur J Endocrinol 157:669–676
101. Legro RS, Barnhart HX, Schlaff WD et al (2007) Clomiphene, metformin, or both for infertility in the polycystic ovary syndrome. N Engl J Med 356:551–566
102. Nawrocka J, Starczewski A (2007) Effects of metformin treatment in women with polycystic ovary syndrome depends on insulin resistance. Gynecol Endocrinol 23:231–237
103. Marcondes JA, Yamashita SA, Maciel GA et al (2007) Metformin in normal-weight hirsute women with polycystic ovary syndrome with normal insulin sensitivity. Gynecol Endocrinol 23:273–278
104. Deplewski D, Rosenfield RL (2000) Role of hormones in pilosebaceous unit development. Endocr Rev 21:363–392
105. Kolodziejczyk B, Duleba AJ et al (2000) Metformin therapy decreases hyperandrogenism and hyperinsulinemia in women with polycystic ovary syndrome. Fertil Steril 73:1149–1154
106. Costello MF, Shrestha B, Eden J et al (2007) Metformin versus oral contraceptive pill in polycystic ovary syndrome: a Cochrane review. Hum Reprod 22:1200–1209
107. Morin-Papunen LC, Vauhkonen I, Koivunen RM et al (2000) Endocrine and metabolic effects of metformin versus ethinyl estradiol-cyproterone acetate in obese women with polycystic ovary syndrome: a randomized study. J Clin Endocrinol Metab 85:3161–3168
108. Gambineri A, Patton L, Vaccina A et al (2006) Treatment with flutamide, metformin, and their combination added to a hypocaloric diet in overweight-obese women with polycystic ovary syndrome: a randomized, 12-month, placebo-controlled study. J Clin Endocrinol Metab 91:3970–3980
109. Al-Ozairi E, Quinton R, Advani A (2008) Therapeutic response to metformin in an underweight patient with polycystic ovarian syndrome. Fertil Steril 90(4):1197.e1–1197.e4
110. Barbieri RL (2007) Clomiphene versus metformin for ovulation induction in polycystic ovary syndrome: the winner is…. J Clin Endocrinol Metab 92:3399–3401
111. Shaw RJ, Lamia KA, Vasquez D et al (2005) The kinase LKB1 mediates glucose homeostasis in liver and therapeutic effects of metformin. Science 310:1642–1646

112. Nestler JE, Jakubowicz DJ (1996) Decreases in ovarian cytochrome P-450c17 alpha activity and serum free testosterone after reduction of insulin secretion in polycystic ovary syndrome. N Engl J Med 335:617–623

113. Panidis D, Tziomalos K, Papadakis E et al (2013) The guidelines issued by the European Society for Human Reproduction and Embryology and the American Society for Reproductive Medicine regarding the induction of ovulation with metformin in patients with the polycystic ovary syndrome potentially require reconsideration. Hormones 12(2): 192–200

114. Palomba S, Orio F Jr, Falbo A et al (2005) Prospective parallel randomized, double-blind, double-dummy controlled clinical trial comparing clomiphene citrate and metformin as the first-line treatment for ovulation induction in nonobese anovulatory women with polycystic ovary syndrome. J Clin Endocrinol Metab 90:4068–4074

115. Tang T, Lord JM, Norman RJ et al (2012) Insulin-sensitising drugs (metformin, rosiglitazone, pioglitazone, D-chiro-inositol) for women with polycystic ovary syndrome, oligo amenorrhoea and subfertility. Cochrane Database Syst Rev (5):CD003053

116. Creanga AA, Bradley HM, McCormick C, Wltkop CT (2008) Uses of metformin in polycystic ovary syndrome: a meta analysis. Obstet Gynecol 111:959–968

117. National Collaborating Centre for women's and children's Health/National Institute for Clinical Excellence (2004) Fertility: assessment and treatment for people with fertility problems, vol 11, Clinical guideline. RCOG Press, London

118. Brown J, Farquhar C, Beck J et al (2009) Clomiphene and anti-oestrogens for ovulation induction in PCOS. Cochrane Database Syst Rev (4):CD002249

119. Vandermolen DT, Ratts VS, Evans WS et al (2011) Metformin increases the ovulatory rate and pregnancy rate from clomiphene citrate in patients with polycystic ovary syndrome who are resistant to clomiphene citrate alone. Fertil Steril 75:310–315

120. Kocak M, Caliskan E, Simsir C et al (2002) Metformin therapy improves ovulatory rates, cervical scores, and pregnancy rates in clomiphene citrate-resistant women with polycystic ovary syndrome. Fertil Steril 77:101–106

121. Malkawi HY, Qublan HS (2002) The effect of metformin plus clomiphene citrate on ovulation and pregnancy rates in clomiphene-resistant women with polycystic ovary syndrome. Saudi Med J 23:663–666

122. Siebert TI, Kruger TF, Steyn DW, Nosarka S (2006) Is the addition of metformin efficacious in the treatment of clomiphene citrate-resistant patients with polycystic ovary syndrome? A structured literature review. Fertil Steril 86:1432–1437

123. La Marca A, Morgante G, Ciotta L et al (1999) Effects of metformin on adrenal steroidogenesis in women with polycystic ovary syndrome. Fertil Steril 72:985–989

124. Billa E, Kapolla N, Nicopoulou SC et al (2009) Metformin administration was associated with a modification of LH, prolactin and insulin secretion dynamics in women with polycystic ovarian syndrome. Gynecol Endocrinol 25:427–434

125. Palomba S, Falbo A, Orio F, Zullo F (2008) Insulin sensitizing agents and reproductive function in polycystic ovary syndrome patients. Curr Opin Obstet Gynecol 20:364–373

126. Fulghesu AM, Villa P, Pavone V et al (1997) The impact of insulin secretion on the ovarian response to exogenous gonadotropins in polycystic ovary syndrome. J Clin Endocrinol Metab 82:644–648

127. Palomba S, Falbo A, La Sala GB (2014) Metformin and gonadotropins for ovulation induction in patients with polycystic ovary syndrome: a systematic review with meta-analysis of randomized controlled trials. Reprod Biol Endocrinol 12:3

128. La Marca A, Morgante G, Palumbo M et al (2002) Insulin-lowering treatment reduces aromatase activity in response to follicle-stimulating hormone in women with polycystic ovary syndrome. Fertil Steril 78(6):1234–1239

129. Glueck CJ, Wang P, Goldenberg N, Sieve-Smith L (2002) Pregnancy outcomes among women with polycystic ovary syndrome with metformin. Hum Reprod 17:2858–2864

130. Lord JM, Flight IH, Norman RJ (2003) Insulin-sensitizing drugs (metformin, troglitazone, rosiglitazone, pioglitazone, D-chiro inositol) for polycystic ovary syndrome. Cochrane Database Syst Rev (3):CD003053

131. Glueck CJ, Phillips H, Cameron D et al (2001) Continuing metformin throughout pregnancy in women with polycystic ovary syndrome appears to safely reduce first-trimester spontaneous abortion: a pilot study. Fertil Steril 75:46–52

132. Palomba S, Orio F Jr, Falbo A et al (2005) Plasminogen activator inhibitor 1 and miscarriage after metformin treatment and laparoscopic ovarian drilling in patients with polycystic ovary syndrome. Fertil Steril 84:761–765

133. Schachter M, Raziel A, Friedler S et al (2003) Insulin resistance in patients with polycystic ovary syndrome is associated with elevated plasma homocysteine. Hum Reprod 18:721–727

134. Diamanti-Kandarakis E, Piperi C et al (2005) Increased levels of serum advanced glycation end-products in women with polycystic ovary syndrome. Clin Endocrinol (Oxf) 62:37–43

135. Orio F Jr, Palomba S, Cascella T (2005) Improvement in endothelial structure and function after metformin treatment in young normal-weight women with polycystic ovary syndrome: results of a 6-month study. J Clin Endocrinol Metab 90:6072–6076

136. Jakubowicz DJ, Seppala M et al (2001) Insulin reduction with metformin increases luteal phase serum glycodelin and insulin-like growth factor-binding protein 1 concentrations and enhances uterine vascularity and blood flow in the polycystic ovary syndrome. J Clin Endocrinol Metab 86:1126–1133

137. Eng GS, Sheridan RA, Wyman A et al (2007) AMP kinase activation increases glucose uptake, decreases apoptosis, and improves pregnancy outcome in embryos exposed to high IGF-I concentrations. Diabetes 65:2228–2234

138. Chi MM, Schlein AL, Moley KH (2000) High insulin-like growth factor 1 (IGF-1) and insulin concentrations trigger apoptosis in the mouse blastocyst via down-regulation of the IGF-1 receptor. Endocrinology 141:1784–1792

139. Samoto T, Maruo T, Matsuo H et al (1993) Altered expression of insulin and insulin-like growth factor-I receptors in follicular and stromal compartments of polycystic ovaries. Endocr J 40:413–424

140. Palomba S, Pasquali R, Orio F, Nestler JE (2008) Clomiphene citrate, metformin or both as first-step approach in treating anovulatory infertility in patients with polycystic ovary syndrome (PCOS): a systematic review and meta-analysis. Clin Endocrinol (Oxf). doi:10.1111/j.1365-2265.2008.03369.x

141. Moll E, Bossuyt PMM, Korevaar JC et al (2006) Effect of clomiphene citrate plus metformin and clomiphene citrate plus placebo on induction of ovulation in women with newly diagnosed polycystic ovary syndrome: randomized double blind clinical trial. BMJ 332:1461–1462

142. Nanovskaya T, Nekhayeva I, Patrikeeva S et al (2006) Transfer of metformin across the dually perfused human placental lobule. Am J Obstet Gynecol 195:1081–1085

143. Kovo M, Haroutiunian S, Feldman N et al (2008) Determination of metformin transfer across the human placenta using a dually perfused ex vivo placental cotyledon model. Eur J Obstet Gynecol Reprod Biol 136:29–33

144. Vanky E, Zahlsen K, Spigsett O et al (2005) Placental passage of metformin in women with polycystic ovary syndrome. Fertil Steril 83:1575–1578

145. Hague WM, Daroven PM, McIntyre D et al (2004) Metformin crosses the placenta: a modulator for fetal insulin resistance? BMJ 327:880–881

146. Charles B, Norris R, Xiao X et al (2006) Population pharmacokinetics of metformin in late pregnancy. Ther Drug Monit 28:67–72

147. Stowers J, Sutherland H (1975) The use of sulfonylureas, biguanides and insulin in pregnancy. In: Sutherland H, Stowers J (eds) Carbohydrate metabolism in pregnancy and the newborn. Churchill Livingstone, Edinburgh, pp 205–220

148. Carlsen SM, Vanky E (2010) Metformin influence on hormone levels at birth, in PCOS mothers and their newborns. Hum Reprod 25(3):786–790

149. Petitti DB (2003) Combination estrogen-progestin oral contraceptives. N Engl J Med 349:1443–1450

150. Gilbert C, Valois M, Koren G (2006) Pregnancy outcome after first-trimester exposure to metformin: a meta-analysis. Fertil Steril 86:658–663

151. Hellmuth E, Damm P, Molsted-Pedersen L (2000) Oral hypoglycemic agents in 118 diabetic pregnancies. Diabet Med 17:507–511

152. Diamanti-Kandarakis E, Christakou CD et al (2010) Metformin: an old medication of new fashion: evolving new molecular mechanisms and clinical implications in polycystic ovary syndrome. Eur J Endocrinol 162:193–212

153. Glueck CJ, Wang P, Kobayashi S et al (2002) Metformin therapy throughout pregnancy reduces the development of gestational diabetes in women with polycystic ovary syndrome. Fertil Steril 77:520–525

154. Norman RJ, Wang JX, Hague W (2004) Should we continue or stop insulin sensitizing drugs during pregnancy? Curr Opin Obstet Gynecol 16:245–250

155. Nawaz FH, Khalid R, Naru T, Rizvi J (2008) Does continuous use of metformin throughout pregnancy improve pregnancy outcomes in women with polycystic ovarian syndrome? J Obstet Gynaecol Res 34(5):832–837

156. Glueck CJ, Goldenberg N, Wang P et al (2004) Metformin during pregnancy reduces insulin, insulin resistance, insulin secretion, weight, testosterone and development of gestational diabetes: prospective longitudinal assessment of women with polycystic ovary syndrome from preconception throughout pregnancy. Hum Reprod 19:510–521

157. Lautatzis ME, Goulis DG, Vrontakis M (2013) Efficacy and safety of metformin during pregnancy in women with gestational diabetes mellitus or polycystic ovary syndrome: a systematic review. Metab Clin Exp 62:1522–1534

158. Niromanesh S, Alavi A, Sharbaf FR et al (2012) Metformin compared with insulin in the management of gestational diabetes mellitus: a randomized clinical trial. Diabetes Res Clin Pract 98(3):422–429

159. Sibai B, Dekker G (2005) Pre-eclampsia. Lancet 365:785–799

160. Forsbach-Sanchez G, Tamez-Perez HE, Vazquez-Lara J (2005) Diabetes and pregnancy. Arch Med Res 36:291–299

161. Maymone AC, Baillargeon JP, Menard J et al (2011) Oral hypoglycemic agents for gestational diabetes mellitus? Expert Opin Drug Saf 10(2):227–238

162. Gardiner SJ, Begg EJ, Kirkpatrick CM, Buckham RB (2004) Metformin therapy and diabetes in pregnancy. Med J Aust 181:174–175

163. Hale TW, Kristensen JH, Hackett LP et al (2002) Transfer of metformin into human milk. Diabetologia 45:1509–1514

164. Briggs GG, Ambrose PJ, Nageotte MP et al (2005) Excretion of metformin into breast milk and the effect on nursing infants. Obstet Gynecol 105:1437–1441

165. Gardiner DJ, Kirkpatrick CM, Begg EJ et al (2003) Transfer of metformin into human milk. Clin Pharmacol Ther 73:71–77

166. Baillargeon JP, Jakubowicz DJ, Iuorno MJ et al (2004) Effects of metformin and rosiglitazone, alone and in combination, in nonobese women with polycystic ovary syndrome and normal indices of insulin sensitivity. Fertil Steril 82:893–902

167. Sahin I, Serter R, Karakurt F et al (2004) Metformin versus flutamide in the treatment of metabolic consequences of non-obese young women with polycystic ovary syndrome: a randomized prospective study. Gynecol Endocrinol 19:115–124

168. Yilmaz M, Biri A, Karakoc A et al (2005) The effects of rosiglitazone and metformin on insulin resistance and serum androgen levels in obese and lean patients with polycystic ovary syndrome. J Endocrinol Invest 28:1003–1008

169. Ortega-Gonzalez C, Luna S, Hernandez L et al (2005) Responses of serum androgen and insulin resistance to metformin and pioglitazone in obese, insulin-resistant women with polycystic ovary syndrome. J Clin Endocrinol Metab 90:1360–1365

170. Harborne LR, Sattar N, Norman JE et al (2005) Metformin and weight loss in obese women with polycystic ovary syndrome: comparison of doses. J Clin Endocrinol Metab 90:4593–4598

171. Crave JC, Fimbel S, Lejeune H et al (1995) Effects of diet and metformin administration on sex hormone-binding globulin, androgens, and insulin in hirsute and obese women. J Clin Endocrinol Metab 80:2057–2062

172. Kiddy DS, Hamilton-Fairley D, Bush A et al (1992) Improvement in endocrine and ovarian function during dietary treatment of obese women with polycystic ovary syndrome. Clin Endocrinol (Oxf) 36:105–111

173. Glueck CJ, Lang JE, Tracy T et al (1999) Contribution of fasting hyperinsulinemia to prediction of atherosclerotic disease status in 293 hyperlipidemic patients. Metabolism 48:1437–1444
174. Pasquali R, Gambineri A, Biscotti D et al (2000) Effect of long-term treatment with metformin added to hypocaloric diet on body composition, fat distribution and androgen and insulin levels in abdominally obese women with and without the polycystic ovary syndrome. J Clin Endocrinol Metab 85:2767–2774
175. Christ-Crain M, Kola B, Lolli F et al (2008) AMP-activated protein kinase mediates glucocorticoid-induced metabolic changes: a novel mechanism in Cushing's syndrome. FASEB J 22:1672–1683
176. Fukuhara A, Matsuda M, Nishizawa M et al (2005) Visfatin: a protein secreted by visceral fat that mimics the effect of insulin. Science 307:426–430
177. Ozkaya M, Cakal E, Ustun Y et al (2010) Effect of metformin on serum visfatin levels in patients with polycystic ovary syndrome. Fertil Steril 93(3):880–884
178. Yasmin E, Glanville J, Barth J, Balen A (2011) Effect of dose escalation of metformin on clinical features, insulin sensitivity and androgen profile in polycystic ovary syndrome. Eur J Obstet Gynecol Reprod Biol 156:67–71
179. Bruno RV, Pinto de Avila MA, Neves FB et al (2007) Comparison of two doses of metformin (2.5 and 1.5 g/day) for the treatment of polycystic ovary syndrome and their effect on body mass index and waist circumference. Fertil Steril 88(2):510–512
180. Buchanan TA, Xiang AH, Peters RK et al (2002) Preservation of pancreatic beta-cell function and prevention of type 2 diabetes by pharmacological treatment of insulin resistance in high-risk Hispanic women. Diabetes 51:2796–2803
181. Salley KE, Wickham EP, Cheang KI et al (2007) Glucose intolerance in polycystic ovary syndrome: a position statement of the Androgen Excess Society. J Clin Endocrinol Metab 92:4546–4556
182. Meyer C, McGrath BP, Teede HJ (2007) Effects of medical therapy on insulin resistance and the cardiovascular system in polycystic ovary syndrome. Diabetes Care 30:471–478
183. Zimmermann S, Philips RA, Dunaif A et al (1992) Polycystic ovary syndrome: lack of hypertension despite profound insulin resistance. J Clin Endocrinol Metab 75:508–513
184. Elting MW, Korsen TJM et al (2001) Prevalence of diabetes mellitus, hypertension and cardiac complaints in a follow-up study of a Dutch PCOS population. Hum Reprod 16:556–560
185. Topcu S, Tok D, Caliskan M et al (2006) Metformin therapy improves coronary microvascular function in patients with polycystic ovary syndrome and insulin resistance. Clin Endocrinol (Oxf) 65:75–80
186. Lord JM, Flight IH, Norman RJ (2003) Metformin in polycystic ovary syndrome: systematic review and meta-analysis. BMJ 327:951–953
187. Glueck CJ, Wang P, Fontaine R et al (1999) Metformin-induced resumption of normal menses in 39 of 43 (91%) previously amenorrheic women with polycystic ovary syndrome. Metabolism 48:511–519
188. Mather KJ, Kwan F, Corenblum B (2000) Hyperinsulinemia in polycystic ovary syndrome correlates with increased cardiovascular risk independent of obesity. Fertil Steril 73:150–156
189. Cibula D, Cifkova R, Fanta M et al (2000) Increased risk of non-insulin dependent diabetes mellitus, arterial hypertension, and coronary artery disease in perimenopausal women with a history of the polycystic ovary syndrome. Hum Reprod 15:787–789
190. Amowitz LL, Sobel BE (1999) Cardiovascular consequences of polycystic ovary syndrome. Endocrinol Metab Clin North Am 28:439–458
191. Birdsall MA, Farquhar CM, White HD (1997) Association between polycystic ovaries and extent of coronary artery disease in women having cardiac catheterization. Ann Intern Med 126:32–35
192. Pasquali R, Filicori M (1998) Insulin sensitizing agents and polycystic ovary syndrome. Eur J Endocrinol 138:253–254
193. Rizzo M, Berneis K, Carmina E, Rini GB (2008) How should we manage atherogenic dyslipidemia in women with polycystic ovary syndrome? Am J Obstet Gynecol 198:28.e1–28.e5
194. Cheang KI, Huszar JM, Best AM et al (2009) Long-term effect of metformin on metabolic parameters in the polycystic ovary syndrome. Diab Vasc Dis Res 6(2):110–119

195. Glueck CJ, Aregawi D, Agloria M et al (2006) Sustainability of 8% weight loss, reduction of insulin resistance, and amelioration of atherogenic-metabolic risk factors over 4 years by metformin-diet in women with polycystic ovary syndrome. Metabolism 55:1582–1589

196. Morin-Papunen LC, Rautio K, Ruokonen A et al (2003) Metformin reduces serum C-reactive protein levels in women with polycystic ovary syndrome. J Clin Endocrinol Metab 88:4649–4654

197. Isoda K, Young JL, Zirlik A et al (2006) Metformin inhibits proinflammatory responses and nuclear factor-kB in human vascular wall cells. Arterioscler Thromb Vasc Biol 26:611–617

198. Shimbo D, Grahame-Clarke C, Miyake Y et al (2007) The association between endothelial dysfunction and cardiovascular outcomes in a population-based multi-ethnic cohort. Atherosclerosis 192:197–203

199. Rossi R, Nuzzo A, Origliani G, Modena MG (2008) Prognostic role of flow-mediated dilation and cardiac risk factors in post-menopausal women. J Am Coll Cardiol 51:997–1002

200. Naka KK, Kalantaridou SN, Kravariti M et al (2011) Effect of the insulin sensitizers metformin and pioglitazone on endothelial function in young women with polycystic ovary syndrome: a prospective randomized study. Fertil Steril 95(1):203–209

201. Ozgurtas T, Oktenli C, Dede M et al (2008) Metformin and oral contraceptive treatments reduced circulating asymmetric dimethylarginine (ADMA) levels in patients with polycystic ovary syndrome (PCOS). Atherosclerosis 200:336–344

202. Teede HJ, Meyer C, Hutchison SK et al (2010) Endothelial function and insulin resistance in polycystic ovary syndrome: the effects of medical therapy. Fertil Steril 93(1):184–209

203. Banfi C, Eriksson P, Giandomenico G et al (2001) Transcriptional regulation of plasminogen activator inhibitor type 1 gene by insulin: insights into the signaling pathway. Diabetes 50:1522–1530

204. Kooistra T, Bosma PJ, Tons HA et al (1989) Plasminogen activator inhibitor 1: biosynthesis and mRNA level are increased by insulin in cultured human hepatocytes. Thromb Haemost 62:723–728

205. Schneider DJ, Nordt TK, Sobel BE (1992) Stimulation by proinsulin of expression of plasminogen activator inhibitor type-I in endothelial cells. Diabetes 41:890–895

206. Morteza Taghavi S, Rokni H, Fatemi S (2011) Metformin decreases thyrotropin in overweight women with polycystic ovarian syndrome and hypothyroidism. Diab Vasc Dis Res 8(1):47–48

207. Janssen OE, Mehlmauer N, Hahn S et al (2004) High prevalence of autoimmune thyroiditis in patients with polycystic ovary syndrome. Eur J Endocrinol 150:363–369

208. Vigersky RA, Filmore-Nassar A, Glass AR (2006) Thyrotropin suppression by metformin. J Clin Endocrinol Metab 91:225–227

209. Cappelli C, Rotondi M, Pirola I et al (2009) TSH-lowering effect of metformin in type 2 diabetes. Diabetes Care 32:1589–1590

210. Ortega-Gonzalez C, Cardoza L, Coutino B et al (2005) Insulin sensitizing drugs increase the endogenous dopaminergic tone in obese insulin-resistant women with polycystic ovary syndrome. J Endocrinol 184:233–239

211. Quigley ME, Rakoff JS, Yen SSC (1981) Increased luteinizing hormone sensitivity to dopamine inhibition in polycystic ovary syndrome. J Clin Endocrinol Metab 52:231–234

212. Nestler JE, Jakubowicz DJ (1997) Lean women with polycystic ovary syndrome respond to insulin reduction with decreases in ovarian P450c17α activity and serum androgens. J Clin Endocrinol Metab 82:4075–4079

213. Iuorno M, Nestler J (1999) The polycystic ovary syndrome: treatment with insulin sensitizing agents. Diabetes Obes Metab 1:127–136

214. Sahin Y, Unluhizarcit K, Yilmazsoy A et al (2007) The effects of metformin on metabolic and cardiovascular risk factors in nonobese women with polycystic ovary syndrome. Clin Endocrinol 67:904–908

215. Kjotrod SB, Carlsen SM, Rasmussen PE et al (2011) Use of metformin before and during assisted reproductive technology in non-obese young infertile women with polycystic ovary

syndrome: a prospective, randomized, double-blind, multi-centre study. Hum Reprod 26(8):2045–2053

216. Trent M, Rich M, Austin SB et al (2001) Society for adolescent medicine: quality of life in girls with polycystic ovary syndrome. J Adolesc Health 28(2):99

217. Pasquali R, Antenucci D, Casimirri F et al (1989) Clinical and hormonal characteristics of obese amenorrheic hyperandrogenic women before and after weight loss. J Clin Endocrinol Metab 68(1):173

218. Hsia Y, Dawoud D, Sutcliffe AG et al (2011) Unlicensed use of metformin in children and adolescents in the UK. Br J Clin Pharmacol 73(1):135–139

219. Ibanez L, Ferrer A, Ong K et al (2004) Insulin sensitization early after menarche prevents progression from precocious pubarche to polycystic ovary syndrome. J Pediatr 144:23–29

220. Bredella MA, McManust S, Misra M (2013) Impact of metformin monotherapy versus metformin with oestrogen-progesterone on lipids in adolescent girls with polycystic ovarian syndrome. Clin Endocrinol 79:199–203

221. Geller DH, Pacaud D, Gordon CM et al (2011) State of the art review: emerging therapies: the use of insulin sensitizers in the treatment of adolescents with polycystic ovary syndrome (PCOS). Int J Pediatr Endocrinol 2011:9

222. Givens JR, Anderse RN, Wiser WL et al (1974) Dynamics of suppression and recovery of plasma FSH, LH, androstenedione and testosterone in polycystic ovarian disease using an oral contraceptive. J Clin Endocrinol Metab 38:727–735

223. Mastorakos G, Koliopoulos C, Creatsas G (2002) Androgen and lipid profiles in adolescents with polycystic ovary syndrome who were treated with two forms of combined oral contraceptives. Fertil Steril 77:919–927

224. Mastorakos G, Koliopoulos C, Deligeoroglou E et al (2006) Effects of two forms of combined oral contraceptives on carbohydrate metabolism in adolescents with polycystic ovary syndrome. Fertil Steril 85:420–427

225. Ibanez L, Lopez-Bermejo A, del Rio L et al (2007) Combined low-dose pioglitazone, flutamide, and metformin for women with androgen excess. J Clin Endocrinol Metab 92:1710–1714

226. Glueck CJ, Moreira A, Goldenberg N et al (2003) Pioglitazone and metformin in obese women with polycystic ovary syndrome not optimally responsive to metformin. Hum Reprod 18:1618–1625

227. Farnier M, Davignon J (1998) Current and future treatment of hyperlipidemia: the role of statins. Am J Cardiol 82:3J–10J

228. Scandinavian Simvastatin Survival Study (4S) (1994) Randomised trial of cholesterol lowering in 4444 patients with coronary heart disease. Lancet 344:1383–1389

229. Clearfield M (2003) Evolution of cholesterol management therapies: exploiting potential for further improvement. Am J Ther 10:275–281

230. McFarlane SI, Muniyappa R, Francisco R, Sowers JR (2002) Pleiotropic effects of statins: lipid reduction and beyond. J Clin Endocrinol Metab 87:1451–1458

231. Banaszewska B, Pawelczyk L, Spaczynski R et al (2011) Effects of simvastatin and metformin on polycystic ovary syndrome after six months of treatment. J Clin Endocrinol Metab 96(11):3493–3501

232. Gao L, Zhao FL, Li SC (2012) Statin is a reasonable treatment option for patients with polycystic ovary syndrome: a meta-analysis of randomized controlled trials. Exp Clin Endocrinol Diabetes 120:367–375

233. Kazerooni T, Shojaei-Baghini S, Dehbashi S et al (2010) Effects of metformin plus simvastatin on polycystic ovary syndrome: a prospective, randomized, double-blind, placebo-controlled study. Fertil Steril 94(6):2208–2213

234. Izquierdo D, Foyouzi N, Kwintkiewicz J et al (2004) Mevastatin inhibits ovarian theca-interstitial cell proliferation and steroidogenesis. Fertil Steril 82(Suppl 3):1193–1197

235. Wu CH, Chen YF, Wan JY et al (2002) Mutant K-ras oncogene regulates steroidogenesis of normal human adrenocortical cells by the RAF-MEK-MAPK pathway. Br J Cancer 87:1000–1005

236. Wu CH, Lee SC, Chiu HH et al (2002) Morphologic change and elevation of cortisol secretion in cultured human normal adrenocortical cells caused by mutant p21K-ras protein. DNA Cell Biol 21:21–29
237. Rzepczynska IJ, Piotrowski PC, Wong DH et al (2009) Role of isoprenylation in simvastatin-induced inhibition of ovarian theca-interstitial growth in the rat. Biol Reprod 81:850–855
238. Bozdag G, Yildiz BO (2013) Interventions for the metabolic dysfunction in polycystic ovary syndrome. Steroids 78:777–781
239. Holub BJ (1986) Metabolism and function of myo-inositol and inositol phospholipids. Annu Rev Nutr 6:563–597
240. Schlemmer U, Frolich W, Prieto RM, Grases F (2009) Phytate in foods and significance for humans: food sources, intake, processing, bioavailability, protective role and analysis. Mol Nutr Food Res 53:S330–S375
241. Croze ML, Soulage CO (2013) Potential role and therapeutic interests of myo-inositol in metabolic disease. Biochimie 95:1811–1827
242. Eagle H, Oyama VI, Levy M, Freeman A (1956) Myo-inositol as an essential growth factor for normal and malignant human cells in tissue culture. Science 123:845–847
243. Chau JFL, Lee MK, Law JWS et al (2005) Sodium/myo inositol cotransporter-1 is essential for the development and function of the peripheral nerves. FASEB 19:1887–1889
244. Dai Z, Chung SK, Miao D et al (2011) Sodium/myoinositol cotransporter 1 and myo-inositol are essential for osteogenesis and bone formation. J Bone Miner Res 26:582–590
245. Deranieh RM, Greenberg ML (2009) Cellular consequences of inositol depletion. Biochem Soc Trans 37:1099–1103
246. Jones DR, Varela-Niero I (1999) Diabetes and the role of inositol-containing lipids in insulin signaling. Mol Med 5:505–514
247. Larner J, Brautigan DL, Thorner MO (2010) D-Chiro-inositol glycans in insulin signaling and insulin resistance. Mol Med 16:543–552
248. Saltiel AR (1990) Second messengers of insulin action. Diabetes Care 13:244–256
249. Pak Y, Paule CR, Bao YD et al (1993) Insulin stimulates the biosynthesis of chiro-inositol-containing phospholipids in a rat fibroblast line expressing the human insulin receptor. Proc Natl Acad Sci U S A 90:7759–7763
250. Chang HG (2011) Mechanisms underlying the abnormal inositol metabolisms in diabetes mellitus. Thesis, Research Space@Auckland
251. Asplin I, Galasko G, Larner J (1993) Chiro-inositol deficiency and insulin resistance: a comparison of the chiro-inositol- and the myo-inositol-containing insulin mediators isolated from urine, hemodialysate, and muscle of control and type II diabetic subjects. Proc Natl Acad Sci 90(13):5924–5928
252. Colazingari S, Treglia M, Najjar R, Bevilacqua A (2013) The combined therapy myo-inositol plus D-chiro-inositol, rather than D-chiro-inositol, is able to improve IVF outcomes: results from a randomized controlled trial. Arch Gynecol Obstet 288:1405–1411
253. Larner J (2002) D-chiro-inositol – its functional role in insulin action and its deficit in insulin resistance. Int J Exp Diabetes Res 3(1):47–60
254. Larner J, Craig JW (1996) Urinary myo-inositol-to-chiro-inositol ratios and insulin resistance. Diabetes Care 19:76–78
255. Pak Y, Huang LC, Lilley KJ, Larner J (1992) In vivo conversion of [3H]myo-inositol to [3H] chiroinositol in rat tissue. J Biol Chem 267:16904–16910
256. Baillargeon J-P, Diamanti-Kandarakis E, Nestler JE et al (2006) Altered D-chiro-inositol urinary clearance in women with polycystic ovary syndrome. Diabetes Care 29(2):300–305
257. Baillargeon JP, Iuorno MJ, Apridonidze T, Nestler J (2010) Uncoupling between insulin and release of a D-chiro-inositol-containing inositolphosphoglycan mediator of insulin action in obese women with polycystic ovary syndrome. Metab Syndr Relat Disord 8(2):127–135
258. Nestler JE, Jakubowicz DJ, Baillargeon JP et al (1999) Ovulatory and metabolic effects of D-chiro-inositol in the polycystic ovary syndrome. N Engl J Med 340:1314–1320
259. Iuorno MJ, Jakubowicz DJ, Baillargeon JP et al (2002) Effects of D-chiro-inositol in lean women with the polycystic ovary syndrome. Endocr Pract 8:417–423

260. Gerli S, Mignosa M, Di Renzo GC (2003) Effects of inositol on ovarian function and metabolic factors in women with PCOS: a randomized double blind placebo-controlled trial. Eur Rev Med Pharmacol Sci 7:151–159

261. Papaleo E, Unfer V, Baillargeon JP et al (2009) Myo-inositol may improve oocyte quality in intracytoplasmic sperm injection cycles. A prospective, controlled, randomized trial. Fertil Steril 91:1750–1754

262. Papaleo E, Unfer V, Baillargeon JP et al (2007) Myo-inositol in patients with polycystic ovary syndrome: a novel method for ovulation induction. Gynecol Endocrinol 23:700–703

263. Cheang KI, Baillargeon JP, Essah PA et al (2008) Insulin-stimulated release of D-chiro-inositol-containing inositolphosphoglycan mediator correlates with insulin sensitivity in women with polycystic ovary syndrome. Metab Clin Exp 57:1390–1397

264. Genazzani AD, Prati A, Santagni S et al (2012) Differential insulin response to myo-inositol administration in obese polycystic ovary syndrome patients. Gynecol Endocrinol 28(12):969–973

265. Genazzani AD, Lanzoni C, Ricchieri F, Jasonni V (2008) Myo-inositol administration positively affects hyperinsulinemia and hormonal parameters in overweight patients with polycystic ovary syndrome. Gynecol Endocrinol 24(3):139–144

266. Zacchè M, Caputo L, Filippis S et al (2009) Efficacy of myo-inositol in the treatment of cutaneous disorders in young women with polycystic ovary syndrome. Gynecol Endocrinol 25(8):508–513

267. Pizzo A, Laganà AS, Barbaro L (2014) Comparison between effects of myo-inositol and D-chiro-inositol on ovarian function and metabolic factors in women with PCOS. Gynecol Endocrinol 30(3):205–208

268. Costantino D, Minozzi G, Minozzi F, Guaraldi C (2009) Metabolic and hormonal effects of myo-inositol in women with polycystic ovary syndrome: a double blind trial. Eur Rev Med Pharmacol Sci 13:105–110

269. Gerli S, Papaleo E, Ferrari A, Di Renzo GC (2007) Randomized, double blind placebo-controlled trial: effects of myo-inositol on ovarian function and metabolic factors in women with PCOS. Eur Rev Med Pharmacol Sci 11(5):347–354

270. Ciotta L, Stracquadanio M, Formuso C et al (2012) D-Chiro-inositol treatment in patients with polycystic ovary syndrome. G Ital Ost Ginecol 34(1):145–148

271. Stracquadanio M, Formuso C, Palumbo MA, Ciotta L (2013) PCOS treatment with an oral contraceptive containing Drospirenone, alone or in association with D-chiro-inositol. G Ital Ost Ginecol 35(4):635–640

272. Carlomagno G, Unfer V (2011) Inositol safety: clinical evidences. Eur Rev Med Pharmacol Sci 15:931–936

273. D'Anna R, Di Benedetto V, Rizzo P et al (2012) Myo-inositol may prevent gestational diabetes in PCOS women. Gynecol Endocrinol 28(6):440–442

274. Costantino D, Guaraldi C (2014) Ruolo del D-chiro-inositolo nelle alterazioni del metabolism glucidico in gravidanza. Minerva Ginecol 66:281–291

275. Pesty A, Lefèvre B, Kubiak J et al (1994) Mouse oocyte maturation is affected by lithium via the polyphosphoinositide metabolism and the microtubule network. Mol Reprod Dev 38:187–199

276. DeLisle S, Blondel O, Longo FJ et al (1996) Expression of inositol 1,4,5-trisphosphate receptors changes the Ca2+ signal of Xenopus oocytes. Am J Physiol 270(4 Pt 1):C1255–C1261

277. Carroll J, Jones KT, Whittingham DG (1996) Ca^{2+} release and the development of Ca^{2+} release mechanisms during oocyte maturation: a prelude to fertilization. Rev Reprod 1:137–143

278. Goud PT, Goud AP, Leybaert L et al (2002) Inositol 1,4,5-trisphosphate receptor function in human oocytes: calcium responses and oocyte activation-related phenomena induced by photolytic release of InsP3 are blocked by a specific antibody to the type 1 receptor. Mol Hum Reprod 8:912–918

279. Chiu TT, Rogers MS, Briton-Jones C, Haines C (2003) Effects of myo-inositol on the in-vitro maturation and subsequent development of mouse oocytes. Hum Reprod 18:408–416

280. Unfer V, Carlomagno G, Rizzo P et al (2011) Myo-inositol rather than D-chiro-inositol is able to improve oocyte quality in intracytoplasmic sperm injection cycles. A prospective, controlled, randomized trial. Eur Rev Med Pharmacol Sci 15:452–457

281. Carlomagno G, Unfer V, Roseff S (2011) The D-chiro-inositol paradox in the ovary. Fertil Steril 95:2515–2516
282. Chattopadhayay R, Ganesh A, Samanta J et al (2010) Effect of follicular fluid oxidative stress on meiotic spindle formation in infertile women with polycystic ovarian syndrome. Gynecol Obstet Invest 69:197–202
283. Ciotta L, Stracquadanio M, Pagano I et al (2011) Effects of myo-inositol supplementation on oocyte's quality in PCOS patients: a double blind trial. Eur Rev Med Pharmacol Sci 15:509–514
284. Artini PG, Di Berardino OM, Papini F et al (2013) Endocrine and clinical effects of myo-inositol administration in polycystic ovary syndrome. A randomized study. Gynecol Endocrinol 29(4):375–379
285. Nordio M, Proietti E (2012) The combined therapy with myo-inositol and D-chiro-inositol reduces the risk of metabolic disease in PCOS overweight patients compared to myo-inositol supplementation alone. Eur Rev Med Pharmacol Sci 16:575–581
286. Minozzi M, Nordio M, Pajalich R (2013) The combined therapy myo-inositol plus D-Chiro-inositol, in a physiological ratio, reduces the cardiovascular risk by improving the lipid profile in PCOS patients. Eur Rev Med Pharmacol Sci 17:537–540
287. Palacio JR, Iborra A, Ulcova-Gallova Z et al (2006) The presence of antibodies to oxidative modified proteins in serum from polycystic ovary syndrome patients. Clin Exp Immunol 144:217–222
288. Victor VM, Rocha M, Banuls C et al (2011) Induction of oxidative stress and human leukocyte/endothelial cell interactions in polycystic ovary syndrome patients with insulin resistance. J Clin Endocrinol Metab 96:3115–3122
289. Gonzalez F, Rote NS, Minium J, Kirwan JP (2006) Reactive oxygen species- induced oxidative stress in the development of insulin resistance and hyperandrogenism in polycystic ovary syndrome. J Clin Endocrinol Metab 91:336–340
290. Agarwal A, Aponte-Mellado A, Premkumar BJ et al (2012) The effects of oxidative stress on female reproduction: a review. Reprod Biol Endocrinol 10:49
291. De Leo V, La Marca A, Cappelli V et al (2012) Valutazione del trattamento con D-Chiro-inositolo sui livelli di stress ossidative nelle pazienti con PCOS. Minerva Ginecol 64:6
292. Sugino N (2005) Reactive oxygen species in ovarian physiology. Reprod Med Biol 4:31–44
293. Sugino N (2007) Roles of reactive oxygen species in the corpus luteum. Anim Sci J 77:556–565
294. Yang HW, Hwang KJ, Kwon HC et al (1998) Detection of reactive oxygen species (ROS) and apoptosis in human fragmented embryos. Hum Reprod 13:998–1002
295. Donà G, Sabbadin C, Fiore C et al (2012) Inositol administration reduces oxidative stress in erythrocytes of patients with polycystic ovary syndrome. Eur J Endocrinol 166:703–710
296. Reiter RJ (1991) Pineal melatonin: cell biology of its synthesis and of its physiological interactions. Endocr Rev 12:151–180
297. Yie SM, Brown GM, Liu GY et al (1995) Melatonin and steroids in human pre-ovulatory follicular fluid: seasonal variations and granulosa cell steroid production. Hum Reprod 10:50–55
298. Brzezinski A, Seibel MM, Lynch HJ et al (1987) Melatonin in human preovulatory follicular fluid. J Clin Endocrinol Metab 64:865–867
299. Ronnberg L, Kauppila A, Leppaluoto J et al (1990) Circadian and seasonal variation in human preovulatory follicular fluid melatonin concentration. J Clin Endocrinol Metab 71:492–496
300. Manda K, Ueno M, Anzai K (2007) AFMK a melatonin metabolite, attenuates X-ray induced oxidative damage to DNA, proteins and lipids in mice. J Pineal Res 42:386–393
301. Tan DX, Chen LD, Poeggeler B et al (1993) Melatonin: a potent, endogenous hydroxyl radical scavenger. Endocr J 1:57–60
302. Tan DX, Manchester LC, Terron MP et al (2007) One molecule, many derivatives: a never-ending interaction of melatonin with reactive oxygen and nitrogen species? J Pineal Res 42:28–42

303. Zavodnik IB, Domansky AV, Lapshina EA et al (2006) Melatonin directly scavenges free radicals generated in red blood cells and a cell-free system: chemiluminescence measurements and theoretical calculations. Life Sci 79:391–400

304. Tomas-Zapico C, Coto-Montes A (2005) A proposed mechanism to explain the stimulatory effect of melatonin on antioxidative enzymes. J Pineal Res 39:99–104

305. Rizzo P, Raffone E, Benedetto V (2010) Effect of the treatment with myo-inositol plus folic acid plus melatonin in comparison with a treatment with myo-inositol plus folic acid on oocyte quality and pregnancy outcome in IVF cycles. A prospective, clinical trial. Eur Rev Med Pharmacol Sci 14:555–561

306. Pittas AG, Lau J, Hu FB et al (2007) The role of vitamin D and calcium in type 2 diabetes. A systematic review and meta-analysis. J Clin Endocrinol Metab 92(6):2017e29

307. Zemel MB (2004) Role of calcium and dairy products in energy partitioning and weight management. Am J Clin Nutr 79:907e12

308. Young KA, Engelman CD, Langefeld CD et al (2009) Association of plasma vitamin D levels with adiposity in Hispanic and African Americans. Clin Endocrinol Metab 94(9):3306e13

309. Panidis D, Balaris C, Farmakiotis D et al (2005) Serum parathyroid hormone concentrations are increased in women with polycystic ovary syndrome. Clin Chem 51:1691e7

310. ESHRE/ASRM (2004) Revised 2003 consensus on diagnostic criteria and long-term health risks related to polycystic ovary syndrome. Fertil Steril 81:19e25

311. Firouzabadi R, Aflatoonian A, Modarresi S et al (2012) Therapeutic effects of calcium & vitamin D supplementation in women with PCOS. Complement Ther Clin Pract 18:85–88

312. Elimoglu H, Duran C, Kiyici S et al (2010) The effect of vitamin D replacement therapy on insulin resistance and androgen levels in women with polycystic ovary syndrome. J Endocrinol Invest 33(4):234e8

313. Burton Freeman B (2000) Dietary fiber and energy regulation. J Nutr 130:272S–275S

314. Keithley J, Swanson B (2005) Glucomannan and obesity: a critical review. Altern Ther Health Med 11(6):30–34

315. Martino F et al (2005) Effect of dietary supplementation with glucomannan on plasma total cholesterol and low density lipoprotein cholesterol in hypercholesterolemic children. Nutr Metab Cardiovasc Dis 15:174–180

316. Chearskul S et al (2009) Immediate and long-term effects of glucomannan on total ghrelin and leptin in type 2 diabetes mellitus. Diabetes Res Clin Pract 83(2)

317. Vuksan V et al (2008) Viscosity of fiber preloads affects food intake in adolescents. Nutr Metab Cardiovasc Dis 19(7):498–503.

318. Blundell JE, Burley VJ (1987) Satiation, satiety and the action of fibre on food intake. Int J Obes 11:9–25

319. Priya Sumithran MB et al (2011) Long-term persistence of hormonal adaptations to weight loss. N Engl J Med 365:17

320. De Leo V, Tosti C, Cappelli V et al (2014) Combination inositol and glucomannan in PCOS patients. Minerva Ginecol 66(6):527–533

Erratum to: Chapter 4 in Psychological Implications of PCOS

Agata Ando' and Antonio Maria D'Alessandro

Erratum to:

Chapter 4 in Mariagrazia Stracquadanio, Lilliana Ciotta, Metabolic Aspects of PCOS: Treatment with Insulin Sensitizers. doi:10.1007/978-3-319-16760-2_4.

The co-author information on the chapter opening page of chapter 4 was missing.

Co-authors for this chapter were:

Agata Ando' and Antonio Maria D'Alessandro

The online version of the original chapter can be found under
doi:10.1007/978-3-319-16760-2_4

Agata Ando'
Department of Psychology, University of Torino, Sydney, Italy

Antonio Maria D'Alessandro
Department of Psychology, University of Catania,
Catania, NSW, Italy